TREATMENT IN DERMATOLOGY

Other titles in the *New Clinical Applications* Series:

Dermatology (Series Editor Dr J. Verbov)
Dermatological Surgery
Superficial Fungal Infections
Talking Points in Dermatology – I
Current Concepts in Contact Dermatitis
Talking Points – II

Cardiology (Series Editor Dr D. Longmore)
Cardiology Screening

Rheumatology (Series Editors Dr J.J. Calabro and Dr W. Carson Dick)
Ankylosing Spondylitis

NEW CLINICAL APPLICATIONS DERMATOLOGY

TREATMENT IN DERMATOLOGY

Editor

JULIAN L. VERBOV
JP, MD, FRCP, FIBiol

Consultant Dermatologist
Royal Liverpool Hospital,
Liverpool, UK

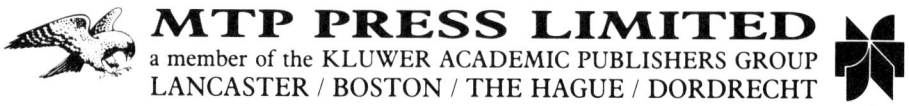

MTP PRESS LIMITED
a member of the KLUWER ACADEMIC PUBLISHERS GROUP
LANCASTER / BOSTON / THE HAGUE / DORDRECHT

Published in the UK and Europe by
MTP Press Limited
Falcon House
Lancaster, England

British Library Cataloguing in Publication Data

Treatment in dermatology.—(New clinical
 applications. Dermatology)
 1. Skin—Diseases
 I. Verbov, Julian II. Series
 616.5′06   RL110

ISBN 0-85200-955-0

Published in the USA by
MTP Press
A division of Kluwer Boston Inc
190 Old Derby Street
Hingham, MA 02043, USA

Library of Congress Cataloging-in-Publication Data

Treatment in dermatology.

 (New clinical applications. Dermatology)
 Includes bibliographies and index.
 1. Skin—Diseases—Treatment. I. Verbov,
Julian. II. Series. [DNLM: 1. Skin Diseases—
therapy. WR 650 T784]
RL110.T74   1987   616.5   86-34270
ISBN 0-85200-955-0

Copyright © 1987 MTP Press Limited

All rights reserved. No part of this publication may be reproduced,
stored in a retrieval system, or transmitted in any form or by any
means, electronic, mechanical, photocopying, recording or otherwise,
without prior permission from the publishers.

Typeset and printed by Butler & Tanner Ltd,
Frome and London

CONTENTS

List of Authors	vi
Series Editor's Foreword	vii
About the Editor	viii
1. Acne *W. J. Cunliffe*	1
2. Leg Ulceration *D. J. Barker*	29
3. Cutaneous Bacterial Infections *A. S. Highet*	63
4. Urticaria *R. P. Warin*	93
5. Psoriasis *T. C. Hindson*	115
Index	137

LIST OF AUTHORS

Dr D. J. Barker, MA, MB, MRCP
Consultant Dermatologist
Bradford Royal Infirmary
Duckworth Lane
Bradford BD9 6RJ

Dr W. J. Cunliffe, MD, FRCP
Consultant Dermatologist
Leeds General Infirmary
Gt. George Street
Leeds LS1 3EX

Dr A. Highet, BSc, MB, MRCP
Consultant Dermatologist
York District Hospital
Wigginton Road
York YO3 7HE

Dr T. C. Hindson, MA, FRCP
Consultant Dermatologist
Sunderland Royal Infirmary
New Durham Road
Sunderland SR2 7JE

Dr R. P. Warin, MD, FRCP
Consultant Dermatologist
Litfield House, 1 Litfield Place
Clifton Down
Bristol BS8 3LS

SERIES EDITOR'S FOREWORD

In this volume I have invited recognized experts to write about everyday problems and their current treatment. The fact that the disorders discussed are common does not make their management any easier. The authors deal in some detail with the many ways in which these conditions present.

I thank all the contributors for their efforts and hope that those who read the book will profit from such expertise.

JULIAN VERBOV

ABOUT THE EDITOR

Dr Julian Verbov is Consultant Dermatologist to Liverpool Health Authority and Clinical Lecturer in Dermatology at the University of Liverpool.

He is a member of the British Association of Dermatologists representing the British Society for Paediatric Dermatology on its Executive Committee. He is a Council Member of the Dermatology Section of the Royal Society of Medicine, and a Member of the North of England Dermatological Society and Editor of its Proceedings.

He is a Fellow of the Zoological Society of London and a Member of the Society of Authors. He is a popular speaker and author of some 180 publications. His special interests include paediatric dermatology, inherited disorders, dermatoglyphics, pruritus ani, therapeutics, and medical humour. He organizes the British Postgraduate Course in Paediatric Dermatology and is a Member of the Editorial Boards of both *Clinical and Experimental Dermatology* and *Pediatric Dermatology*.

1
ACNE

W. J. CUNLIFFE

GENERAL PRINCIPLES

Before considering precisely what to give a patient for the treatment of his/her acne it is necessary to discuss with most patients why they have acne. There are so many myths about acne that it is necessary to squash these myths as well as emphasizing the more important facts.

Many patients these days are less convinced about the link between acne and diet although there are still some diehards who unquestionably believe that animal fats, especially pig fats, will aggravate acne. However available data shows no significant relationship between diet and acne.

Many patients on return from holidays note that their acne is much better. This probably is a genuine biological effect, though the cosmetic camouflage of ultraviolet radiation pigmentation is an important factor plus the fact that when someone is away on holiday even bad things seem better. Studies on the use of artificial ultraviolet radiation are limited but it would appear that frequent visits to a solarium for UVA radiation are of limited help.

The myth that acne is due to an 'infection' still lingers; it is hoped that the physician will bury this myth. Thus, there is no need for the acne patient to wash excessively. There is also belief that makeup will make acne worse; it is likely that the long-term application of heavy makeup could possibly aggravate acne by aggravating poral occlusion. Evidence from the United States of America indicates that certain cosmetics are indeed comedogenic[1]. However a young girl with troublesome acne, psychologically very disturbed, needs some psychological boost and the use of cosmetics to cover inflammatory acne whilst it is in the process of improving is sound advice.

The physician should not underestimate the psychological effect of acne on the individual[2]. The physical and psychological trauma of acne should be well known and a sympathetic approach is essential. There is also a significant incidence of unemployment amongst subjects with clinical acne[3]. Patients, ethnically born with a coloured skin, may produce considerable post-inflammatory pigmentation which can be as disturbing as the active inflammatory lesions.

Many patients have read and seen many advertisements which misguide the patient into thinking that acne responds quickly to treatment. This is not so and must be emphasized to the patient. There is usually no improvement in the first 2–4 weeks, but with appropriate treatment most patients will see 40% improvement at the end of 2 months, 60% improvement at 4 months and 80% or even greater improvement by 6 months.

Total compliance is necessary[4]. Failure to take the tablets correctly and failure to use topical therapy adequately will markedly reduce the rate of response. Certain antibiotics, in particular tetracycline and erythromycin, are less adequately absorbed if taken with food and after food; it is therefore important to take these tablets $\frac{1}{2}$–1 hour before food with a sip of water and not with milk[4].

Patients also have miscomprehensions about topical treatments; they often think that they should only apply the therapy just to the spots. It is important to treat not just the spots but the whole of the sites where the skin is affected.

Most acne patients are otherwise fit and with the possible exception of the contraceptive pill are rarely on other medications. However occasionally a female patient may be taking oral iron tablets for menorrhagia and an older patient with acne may be on antacids for dyspeptic symptoms[5]. Both these preparations will chelate with oral antibiotics; the antacids and iron can be taken after foods, the antibiotics being taken $\frac{1}{2}$–1 hour before foods.

Having made the decision as to the treatment to use and the patient having been given the appropriate advice, a decision has to be taken as to how frequently the patient should be reviewed. In the majority of cases review every 3–4 months is necessary, providing progress is satisfactory. The patient should be given an appointment for 3–4 months but told that if the acne is not responding as well as he/she would like then the patient should make an urgent appointment for review.

The patient must also be told of the treatment side-effects. An irritant dermatitis is common with most topical acne preparations and the severity of this can be controlled by adjusting the frequency of use of the topical therapy[6]. Side-effects of oral antibiotics are uncommon, but include diarrhoea, abdominal colic and vaginal candidiasis[4].

Ideally any physician treating acne should use a grading scale to assess the progress. A practitioner will monitor the treatment of hypertension by measuring the blood pressure; diabetes is monitored by checking the urine for sugar and blood sugar levels. There is no reason why the skin, visible to all, cannot be graded[7]. Figures 1.1–1.4 demonstrate various severities of acne and it is hoped that the physician will use this and other similar guides as a guide to the patient's response.

TOPICAL TREATMENT

It is essential to stress to the patient that topical therapies will need to be used for several years and the application must not just be applied to the spots but to the whole of the affected areas prone to acne, not necessarily just on the face but where appropriate to the back and chest. In this section the major types of acne therapies used topically will be discussed such as benzoyl peroxide[6], retinoic acid[8] and topical antibiotics[9], along with a miscellaneous group, including their availability, formulation and mechanism of action.

Benzoyl peroxide

Benzoyl peroxide has been available for at least 21 years for the treatment of acne. It is available in concentrations of 2.5, 5, 10 and 20% as creams and gels and more recently in the United Kingdom as a wash[4,6].

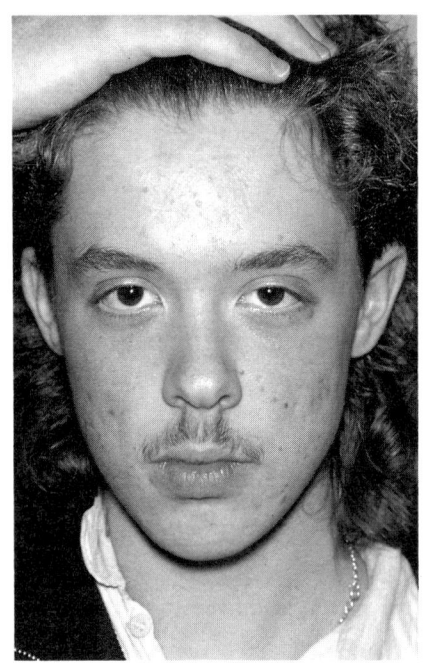

FIGURE 1.1 A patient with facial grade 1.0

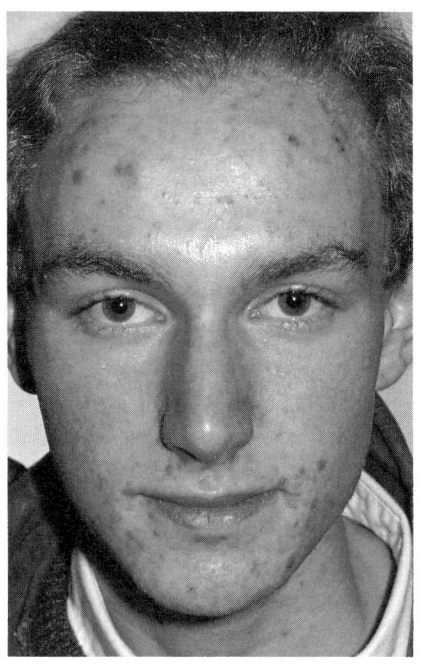

FIGURE 1.2 A patient with facial grade 2.0

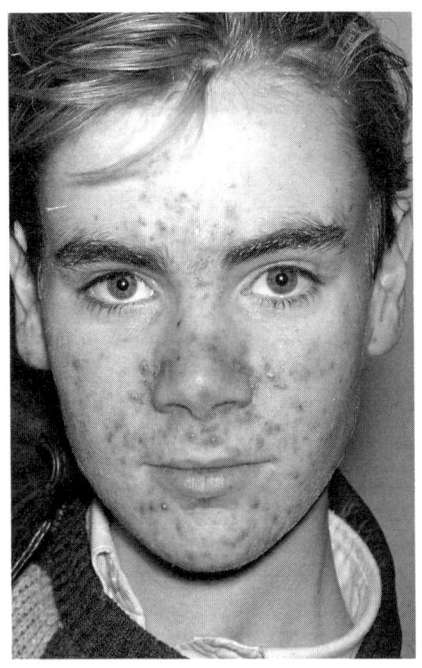

FIGURE 1.3 A patient with facial grade 3.0

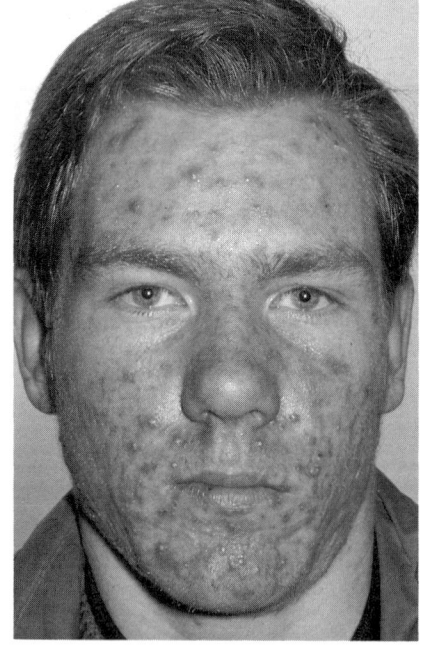

FIGURE 1.4 A patient with facial grade 5.0

Benzoyl peroxide was probably the first proven effective topical treatment for acne vulgaris[10]. Unfortunately there are no suitable dose response studies indicating an increased effectiveness of even the 20% over a 2.5% concentration. It is assumed, without proof, that there may be a dose response effect. However, the prescribing of a higher concentration of benzoyl peroxide is of psychological benefit in a patient whose acne is not doing too badly and in whom the doctor does not wish – as yet – to give oral therapy; thus the physician can play games with the patient and indicate that by increasing the strength of the benzoyl peroxide that this higher concentration could work better.

There are four main aetiological factors responsible for the development of acne lesions[11]. An increased sebum production, comedogenesis, microbial colonization of the pilosebaceous duct and the production of inflammation. The effect of benzoyl peroxide on sebum excretion is questionable. It has been suggested that it has no effect on sebum production but it has been shown by Fanta[12] that it will reduce sebum synthesis.

On the contrary Cunliffe *et al.*[13] showed that benzoyl peroxide may increase sebum excretion rate by up to 16%. These latter authors emphasized that it is unlikely that the drug has a direct effect on sebum production but by reducing comedogenesis may affect the outflow of sebum and so produce an apparent increase.

Studies on the effect of benzoyl peroxide on comedogenesis – using the follicular cast model which gives a reasonable measure of the number of microcomedones – shows that benzoyl peroxide has only a slight effect of the order of about 10%[14]. This figure is similar to the effects of placebo.

Benzoyl peroxide has a dramatic effect reducing by 2 log cycles the number of skin surface *Propionibacterium acnes* and *Staphylococcus epidermidis*[15]. Limited work on ductal bacteria also confirms that benzoyl peroxide reduces colonization in the duct. Although it is no longer accepted that free fatty acids are important in the development of acne, the measurement of skin surface free fatty acids is a good marker of bacterial function. The free fatty acids arise by hydrolysis of sebaceous triglycerides by *P. acnes* and *S. epidermidis*. Benzoyl peroxide in doses of 2.5, 5 and 10% have been shown to produce suppression of skin surface free fatty acids by the order of 40–50%.

Retinoic acid

Retinoic acid[8], like benzoyl peroxide, has been available for at least 20 years, initially as an ointment which was unsuitable for patients with acne but in the last 15 years as highly acceptable cosmetic preparations. The drug is especially helpful in reducing the number of non-inflamed lesions. This has been shown in clinical studies and by using the follicular cast technique as a measure of the number of microcomedones[14]. Since non-inflamed lesions are responsible for the development of inflamed lesions retinoic acid subsequently suppresses the number of inflamed lesions. The mechanism of the drug has been studied predominantly in terms of its role in influencing comedogenesis.

Topical antibiotics

Topical antibiotics are used widely in the USA where there are several brand names of erythromycin, tetracycline and one of clindamycin[9]. Also in several European countries there are several topical antibiotics for the treatment of acne. In England the topical anti-acne antibiotics are chloramphenicol, neomycin and tetracycline. Chloramphenicol is bacteriostatic for *P. acnes* but neomycin has no effect whatsoever on *P. acnes*; so why Neomedone helps (if it does) subjects with acne is a mystery. Recently tetracycline has become available in the UK as a 0.22% lotion. There are few studies comparing non-antibiotic and antibiotic topical acne therapies; one study suggested erythromycin and benzoyl peroxide as equivalent[16]. In another study benzoyl peroxide was superior to chloramphenicol (available as in Actinac)[17].

The mechanism of action of topical antibiotics is predominantly antimicrobial. This is especially so with clindamycin which has been shown to reduce significantly both the number of surface and ductal counts of *P. acnes*[16]. The effect of topical antibiotics on follicular casts has not been investigated; however, clinical enumeration of lesions shows a significant reduction in the number of comedones.

Azelaic acid

Azelaic acid is a dicarboxylic acid derived from *P. ovale*; a few years ago it was discovered, possibly by chance, to be beneficial in acne[18]. Italian[18] and English[19] authors have demonstrated in open studies that the drug can be very effective in acne, even in very severe acne; in Leeds we have demonstrated that the drug is indeed effective, almost as effective as tetracycline.

Azelaic acid reduces free fatty acids by the order of 20% but this effect could be less than real since the azelaic acid itself is a fatty acid and will be sampled when collecting the skin surface lipids[19]. Azelaic acid reduces *P. acnes* by 1 log cycle; this is less than that seen with benzoyl peroxide but of the same order as that seen with oral tetracycline 1 g/day.

Sulphur

This is a time-honoured preparation and has been used in the treatment of acne for at least 40 years[20]. It now achieves much less therapeutic interest because of the availability of more cosmetically elegant, less odiferous, topical therapies and the wider use of oral therapies. It is assumed that the drug predominantly is comedolytic but there is one study that has shown that the drug is possibly even comedogenic.

Anti-androgens

Ever since it was known that acne is an androgen-mediated disorder considerable effort has been made by dermatologists and the drug industry into the development of an active topical anti-androgen which has no systemic effect[21]. There have been many studied in man but on the whole these have been disappointing. Although some preparations in certain bases have been shown in a small number of patients to have some anti-seborrhoeic effect the fact that there is not a suitable one is confirmed by the observation that there is not yet a commercially available preparation. An anti-androgen may not be the most effective drug; a metabolite could be more relevant. The formulation may not penetrate the sebaceous system adequately; certain cutaneous microflora could metabolize and so inactivate the drug.

ORAL THERAPY

Oral treatment is indicated in those subjects with moderate and severe acne. It is also used in those patients with mild acne who are psychologically very depressed and in those in whom employment is difficult because of acne, even if the acne is relatively mild.

The three main groups of oral therapy are antibiotics, hormones and retinoids. Antibiotics are usually the first line of oral therapy.

Antibiotics (and co-trimoxazole/trimethoprim)

For some years either 250 mg or 500 mg of tetracycline daily was the dosage of choice and we in Leeds some 15 years ago contributed to this myth on the use of low dose antibiotics in acne. The use of low dose antibiotics in acne should be totally forgotten. It is only in the last four years that some sense has been instilled so as to allow the logical use of oral antibiotics in acne[22,23]. Tetracycline still remains and should remain the number one choice. Erythromycin is also used and certainly would be the drug of choice in a patient sensitive to tetracycline or in a female who is contemplating pregnancy or in the treatment of a pregnant patient who required oral therapy. Co-trimoxazole is occasionally used especially in patients with so-called gram-negative folliculitis. Trimethoprim is a preferred alternative since it has less side effects than co-trimoxazole. Trimethoprim should also be considered not just in patients with Gram-negative folliculitis but in patients non-responsive to tetracycline and erythromycin or in those who are intolerant to such preparations.

Tetracycline

This is the number one choice and like erythromycin must be given ½–1 hour before food with a sip of water and if the patient is on iron or antacids those therapies must be taken with or after food. The practitioner must initially use the cheaper forms of tetracycline such as tetracycline or oxytetracycline. We have shown as will be indicated later, that the recommended dose is 1 g/day[23].

Erythromycin

This has been shown to be as effective as tetracycline. It is less affected by food and in those individuals where the taking of tablets ½–1 hour before food is impossible, as is occasionally the case, then erythromycin would be the choice.

Minocycline

This brand name of tetracycline – minocycline – is very well absorbed compared to ordinary tetracycline and can be taken with food. The drug may have a quicker effect in the resolution of certain acne lesions and has a greater affect on skin surface *P. acnes*. In controlled studies in the 'average' acne patient, it is *no better* than 1 g of tetracycline (in a dosage of either 100–200 mg/day). It should be considered in a patient not responding to conventional therapy. It is expensive.

Trimethoprim

Studies have shown this to be as good as tetracycline in the average acne patient and limited personal observations – but totally uncontrolled – indicate it to be as effective as co-trimoxazole in Gram-negative folliculitis.

Mechanism of action
The mechanism of action of antibiotics is primarily an antimicrobial one. Doses of 1 g tetracycline/erythromycin will suppress the numbers of *P. acnes* by 1 log cycle, and their function, as indicated by their reduction in surface free fatty acids by up to 50%. This reduction in *P. acnes* numbers is not as large as that produced with benzoyl peroxide; it is quite likely that an important mechanism of action of oral antibiotics is through their anti-inflammatory effects. Oral antibiotics reduce chemotaxis and modify the alternate and classical complement pathways.

HORMONAL REGIMES

There are three major types of hormonal therapy to be considered, oestrogen plus prednisolone[24], oestrogen plus cyproterone acetate[25, 26], and spironolactone[27]. Hormonal regimes should be given for 6–12 months. As with oral antibiotics the rate of response is slow, there will be no response within the first month and sometimes very little until 6 weeks. Diane is a combination of 50 μg ethinyl oestradiol and 2 mg cyproterone acetate: the rate of improvement with Diane is similar to that of 1 g/day of tetracycline. Although an excellent contraceptive, Diane cannot be prescribed primarily as a contraceptive but is prescribed for the female whose acne is not responding well to conventional therapy or in those females whose contraceptive control is jeopardized as a result of antibiotic-induced diarrhoea.

Another alternative, other things being equal, would be to change the oestrogen content of the contraceptive pill from 30 to 50 μg. Until Diane and Roaccutane were available we treated about 10 patients a year with the combination of a 50 μg oestrogen contraceptive pill with prednisolone 5 mg at night. Given at night prednisolone will suppress adrenal androgens. However Diane is much more convenient for the patient to take and is now a well established treatment for acne in Europe.

In older patients, especially those over the age of 30, with various clinical factors which would detract from giving the contraceptive pill, then there is virtue in the use of spironolactone[27]. In females 100–200 mg will have a dramatic effect on acne and this is associated with a concomitant reduction in the seborrhoea.

Another useful indication for spironolactone is the hirsute female since 100–200 mg spironolactone/day will – albeit slowly – reduce the hirsuties. Diane will not effect hirsuties but Diane plus 100 mg CPA given from the 5–15th day of the cycle will have a beneficial effect after several months, on any concomitant hirsuties.

The mechanism of action of all these hormonal regimes is not entirely certain but effects on both systemic and local modulations of hormones are likely. All regimes have a systemic effect and reduce plasma levels of testosterone, DHA (dehydroepiandrostenedione) and other hormones. There is also possibly a local effect of these regimes. The overall result is a reduction in sebum excretion rate and possibly in comedogenesis.

There is also evidence that oestrogens will modulate lymphocyte function. Thus hormones may therefore modulate the acne inflammation.

RETINOIDS

There have been several badly controlled studies investigating the value of oral vitamin A acid in acne. The balance of view is that it does have a beneficial effect in acne but in doses which produce mucocutaneous toxicity disproportionate to the clinical improvement. It is nowhere as effective as oral antibiotics and not in the same category as isotretinoin. Etretinate is of no benefit in acne.

There have been many studies showing the tremendous value of isotretinoin in alleviating severe acne – not just whilst taking the drug but for many months after stopping therapy[28, 29]. A minimum of 4 months therapy is usually required but 15% of patients require 5–7 months treatment. Doses of 0.1–1.0 mg/kg are all effective. Follow-up studies on the rate of relapse have shown a dose–response effect in that patients given 0.5 mg or less show a relapse more quickly and

TABLE 1.1 The percentage of patients relapsing* after stopping isotretinoin

Dose	Months of treatment				
	6	12	24	36	48
0.1 mg/kg	10	82	2	0	0
0.5 mg/kg	9	11	41	11	5
1.0 mg/kg	3	6	7	3	1

* Relapse indicates the need for oral treatment

need oral therapy – maybe with antibiotics but occasionally with isotretinoin (Table 1.1)[29].

It should be appreciated that only in a small number of patients is the acne totally cured by isotretinoin. In most subjects who have received 1.0 mg/kg no further treatment is needed for 12–15 months – but after about 15 months most subjects require some topical therapy such as benzoyl peroxide to control their now mild or physiological acne.

Side-effects are common, and are described later but it is important that the dosage is not reduced; the patient must treat the side effects, which are troublesome at times.

Mechanism of action

Isotretinoin is the only therapy which affects all four main aetiological factors involved in acne[29, 30]. Doses between 0.1–1.0 mg markedly suppress sebum excretion by 75–95% (Figure 1.5). There is a dose-dependent reduction in comedogenesis as assessed by measuring follicular casts[29] (Figure 1.6). This is associated with electron-microscopic changes; the corneocytes are separated, by the accumulation of an intercellular amyloid like material. The desmosomes are enlarged and vacuolated. Isotretinoin has no direct antimicrobial effect *in vitro* – but by making the skin environment alien there is marked reduction in surface *P. acnes* and *S. epidermidis*. These changes are in excess of that produced by antibiotics and benzoyl peroxide.

ACNE

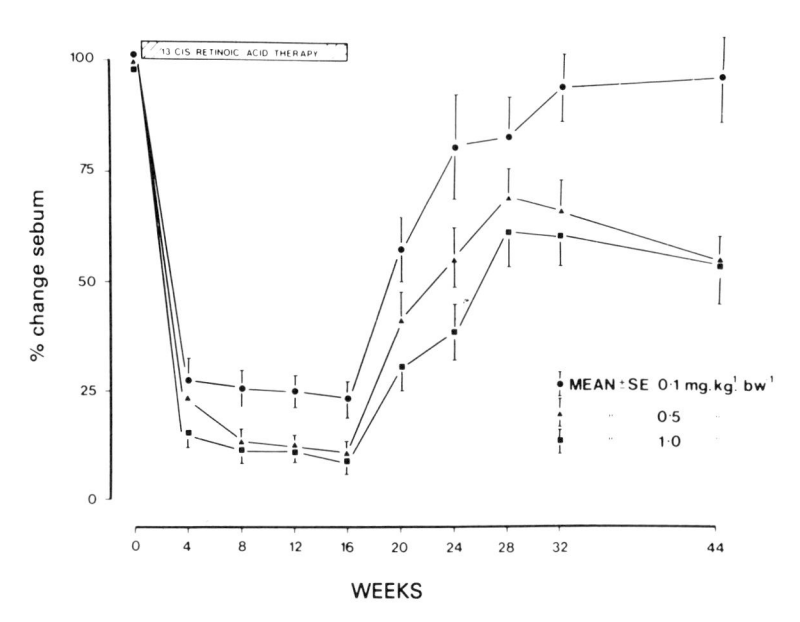

FIGURE 1.5 The dramatic effect of Isotretinoin on Sebum Excretion Rate

There is a relationship between dose, sebum excretion rate (SER) and time off therapy: with doses of 0.1 mg there is a return in most patients to pre-treatment SER within 8–12 months. With 0.5 mg there is a return to almost pre-treatment level by 18 months and in some patients given 1.0 mg this dose maintains a SER 40% of the pre-treatment level even 3 years after stopping therapy. For up to 2 years after stopping therapy patients on 1.0 mg show a significant reduction in follicular casts. On doses of 0.1 and 0.5 mg patients show a return of this measure of comedogenesis to pre-treatment level. After 6–8 months of stopping therapy on all doses the surface bacteria have returned almost towards control level[30].

In vitro it can be demonstrated that isotretinoin suppresses chemotaxis[31] but its *in vivo* significance has not been adequately investigated.

MISCELLANEOUS ORAL THERAPIES

Before anti-androgens and isotretinoin were available the treatment of patients with 'difficult' acne was not easy. Dapsone and Clofazimine

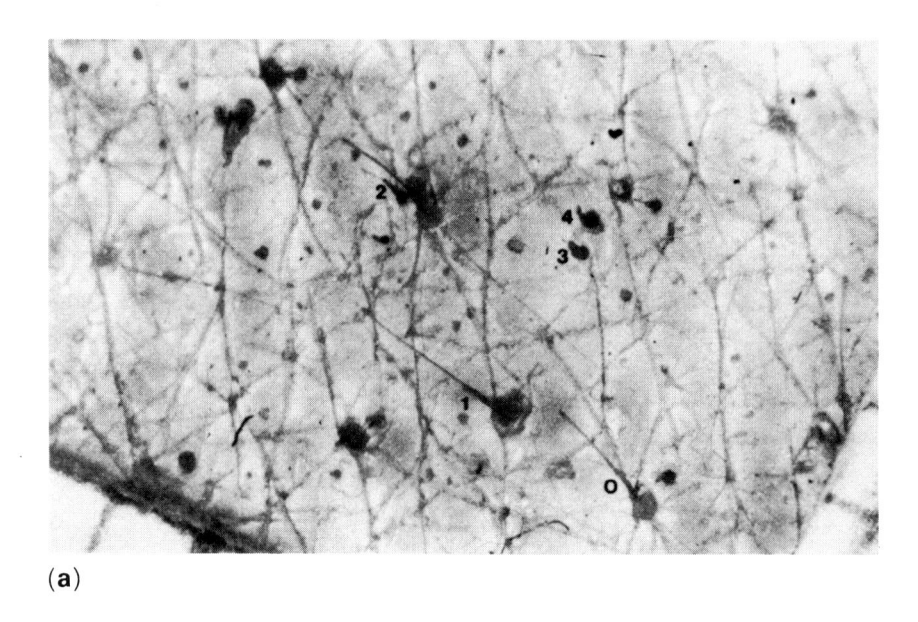

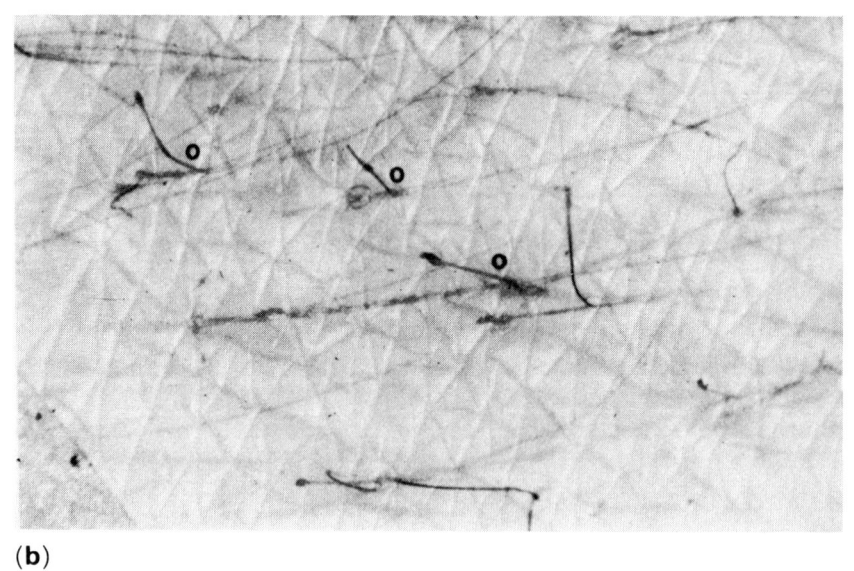

FIGURE 1.6 The effect of Isotretinoin on ductal cornification (**a**) before treatment and (**b**) after treatment

have been reported in non-controlled studies to help. Oral steroids are the drug of choice in acne fulminans. Such patients who develop an immune complex reaction to *P. acnes* present with severe acne – especially on the trunk, fever, polyarthralgia and bone pain. The recommended dosage of prednisolone is 40 mg/day for one week, the dose gradually being reduced to zero over 6 weeks. In addition, the physician often prescribes 1 gm/day of tetracycline or erythromycin.

STRATEGY OF USE

The type of therapy prescribed for a patient with acne depends on the site, severity and type of acne – and the manner in which the patient is responding psychologically to the acne.

It is necessary to reassure the patient that acne is a very treatable disease. The doctor can in no way cure the acne but with long-term treatment the results should be most satisfying. The patient should be told that topical therapy will be necessary for many years and 6–8 month courses of oral therapy may be required. It should be stressed to the patient that treatment of acne is a team affair involving the physician and patient[23].

Treatment of mild acne

Subjects with mild acne should be assessed to determine whether the acne is predominantly inflammatory or non-inflammatory or a mixture. Subjects with predominantly non-inflammatory acne should be given retinoic acid (Retin A). This should be applied once or twice daily to all areas and if appropriate, not just the face but also the back and chest.

If the patient has many obvious blackheads, then the practice nurse or the nurse in dermatological outpatients could remove the blackheads. An intelligent patient could also remove the blackheads but unfortunately both in hospital and in the community the style and type of comedone removers leave much to be desired – at least in the United Kingdom.

If the patient has multiple inflammatory lesions and very few non-inflamed lesions benzoyl peroxide preparations are the drug of choice[32]. The physician should start with a 5% concentration.

Some patients will have mixed non-inflamed and inflamed lesions and such patients can be given Retin A cream in the morning and benzoyl peroxide preparation in the evening. Again if there is any irritant dermatitis they could use one preparation one day and the other the next.

Topical treatment is indicated in three situations (1) those with mild acne, (2) in conjunction with oral therapy – we have shown that combined therapy is better than single therapy and (3) as a maintenance therapy after oral therapy has been discontinued.

Treatment of moderate or severe acne

Certain risk factors dictate the response of the acne patient to therapy[23]. We have shown that in subjects taking 0.5 g/day of erythromycin (plus 5% benzoyl peroxide) that young patients respond less well than old, male patients less well than females, subjects with truncal acne fare less well than those with facial acne, subjects with a greasy skin do less well than those with a less greasy skin and those subjects with a more severe acne respond less well than those with a moderate acne. Based on this information we carried out a study of 250 subjects whereby we demonstrated that if a subject has acne and needs oral therapy there is no justification in giving 0.5 g/day. In this study we demonstrated that with patients matched for age, sex, acne severity and site of acne then those patients receiving 1 g/day showed significantly greater improvement of their acne. 12 months after stopping oral therapy the rate of re-occurrence of the acne was significantly much greater in all subjects, who had received 0.5 g/day. Thus it can be concluded that a subject needing oral therapy should initially receive 1 g/day of tetracycline given as 500 mg twice daily. Although much of our clinical research was based on erythromycin – we chose this therapy as it is better absorbed than oxytetracycline – we have shown no difference in response between oxytetracycline and erythromycin.

If a patient is no better or worse after three months then the oral therapy must be changed. The change could be initially to erythromycin if the patient has been taking tetracycline. If the patient is no better after a further three months another alternative would be one of the brand name tetracyclines such as Doxycycline or Minocycline. These drugs are expensive and put an unnecessary financial load on the health service. It is likely that they are of benefit in patients who are not responding well to conventional therapy; limited studies indicate that this is so but such studies can be criticized on the grounds that they do not adequately define what is meant by failures. The papers quoting the benefit of brand antibiotics state that the patients have failed to respond to conventional therapy without defining what they mean by failure in terms of duration of therapy, dosage and how the therapy was taken.

Trimethoprim is a third alternative but before embarking upon yet another agent good microbiological control is necessary. Thus such a patient should be managed in a hospital clinic since *P. acnes* is notoriously difficult to grow and the problem could be complicated by a Gram-negative folliculitis.

In a female alternative therapy is a hormonal regime. In a female who is sexually active and there are no contra-indications a 50 µg oestrogen pill or Diane could be given for 12 months plus topical therapy. In a female over 30 years or if there are contra-indications to oestrogen therapy, spironolactone 100 mg twice daily can be prescribed.

The really difficult patient

In patients with horrendous acne, or patients whose moderate acne is getting worse despite 3–6 months of therapy and adequate compliance then, whatever the sex, isotretinoin should be given[28,29,33]. This is a hospital only, dermatologist only, prescribable therapy but in the correct situations is unquestionably a most valuable drug. Other indications for isotretinoin are in the patients with moderate acne who have responded well on three occasions to conventional therapy but quickly relapsed on stopping oral therapy. Another group meriting isotretinoin are those patients with severe acne who have responded well but despite all other attempts show an improvement of 50% or less 6–9 months after starting therapy.

WEANING FROM ORAL ANTIBIOTICS

There is no proven clinically scientific way of how best to reduce oral antibiotics. Our policy is a purely empirical one. We tell the patients to gradually reduce the tablets over a period of a month. It should be emphasized to the patient that in no way will the physician allow the acne to return to its pre-antibiotic level of severity and that if necessary the physician would reinstitute therapy with oral antibiotics.

NON-RESPONDERS

The physician must try to determine why the patient has not responded well. Lack of compliance is unquestionably the commonest reason. If a patient has been taking antibiotics regularly then the *S. epidermidis* should be resistant to that antibiotic.

Resistant bacteria (*P. acnes*) are uncommon although both in the United States and in Leeds there is evidence to indicate an increase in resistance to commonly used antibiotics.

An uncommon complication of oral antibiotics is Gram-negative folliculitis[34]. This term is not the best description; in some patients the description fits the title in that the patient suddenly develops crops of multiple pustules. Thus the sudden deterioration of the patient's acne associated with many small superficial pustules should alert the physician to a Gram-negative folliculitis. The organisms involved are usually *E. coli*, *Proteus*, *Pseudomonas* and *Klebsiella* spp. This diagnosis can be confirmed by taking swabs both from the lesions and nose which commonly harbour the organisms.

However the most likely explanation for most patients who fail to respond lies in the way in which the skin handles the drug. On-going research suggests that most of the so-called failures have a very high sebum excretion rate compared to responding subjects.

POST-ACNE SEQUELAE

Some patients develop post-inflammatory scarring and it is the physician's role to appreciate whether this is of concern to the patient. Soft non-fibrotic shallow scars can do well with the injection of bovine collagen (Zyderm)[35]. A test dose read at 6 weeks is given intradermally in the forearm to exclude any hypersensitivity to the bovine collagen; patients with personal or family history of a collagen disease or an immune disease would be precluded from such treatment. Zyderm can only be given at specialized centres.

Dermabrasion in the United Kindom is carried out usually under a general anaesthetic by the plastic surgeon. Dermabrasion should not be recommended if the individual is uncertain whether or not he/she needed the operation. Success is somewhere of the order of 30–80%, the patient's belief of improvement being better than that of the surgeon.

Liquid nitrogen

Acne cysts are cosmetically disfiguring and can be painful especially around the ears or the nose. Such cysts can be treated by the 20-second application of liquid nitrogen – a second treatment being given 2 minutes later[36]. The whole of the cyst must be treated. This therapy works by producing cold damage to the fibrotic cyst wall resulting in chemotaxis of polymorphs whose proteases – hopefully – will subsequently destroy the wall and allow healing. Another treatment for cysts is intralesional injection of triamcinolone[37].

SIDE-EFFECTS OF TREATMENT

The conventional treatment of acne is relatively free of serious side-effects.

Topical treatment

Virtually all topical treatments if used excessively will produce some erythema and some scaling – the so-called primary irritant dermatitis is especially seen around the side of the neck and around the eyes[4, 6]. A moisturizing cream will help this problem and if the problem is excessive a weak steroid ointment such as Haelan (flurandrenalone) ointment will prove beneficial and resolve the dermatitis in a few days. If the problem is recurrent and extensive then patch tests are necessary to exclude an allergic dermatitis either to the active medicament or its base; an allergic dermatitis to benzoyl peroxide is of the order of 1 in 500. Benzoyl peroxide will also occasionally bleach the hair and clothes.

Oral antibiotic treatment

Nausea is extremely uncommon and vomiting is rare. Relatively trivial abdominal colic occurs in 5.2% of patients[4]; this is usually intermittent and often needs no treatment. Should it require treatment Lomotil one tablet twice daily for 1–5 days repeated if necessary usually controls this without a reduction in antibiotic dosage. Vaginal candidiasis occurs in 3.7% but only in sexually active females[4]. Appropriate treatment of the whole gastro-intestinal tract of both partners should be carried out if relevant.

Unusual complications occur. Onycholysis, often painful, is seen occasionally with tetracycline as is oesophagitis. A more common but still infrequent complication occurring with minocycline and to a much lesser extent with tetracycline is the development of benign intracranial hypertension[38]. Such a patient complains of the varied combination of headaches, drowsiness, loss of concentration and blurred vision. Fortunately the problem is totally reversible. Pigmentation is also seen with minocycline[39]. This presents in two ways; firstly, in and around the acne scars; secondly, as macular pigmentation on the shins. The pigmentation is due to the interaction of the minocycline with iron in the dermis; it is self-limiting and slowly improves within several months of discontinuing the treatment. Yellow discolouration of the teeth is only seen in the deciduous teeth and so tetracyclines should not be given during their development, i.e. before the age of 10 years.

Certain tetracyclines, especially the long acting ones, such as demeclocycline HCL may predispose to photosensitivity rashes including photosensitive lichenoid eruptions.

Oral therapy hormones

Side-effects with Diane are no different than conventional 50 μg pills. Spironolactone is not a contraceptive and this must be emphasized to the patient. Menstrual irregularities occur in about 50% of patients. Menstrual irregularities can sometimes be controlled by reducing the dose from 200 mg/day to 150 or 100 mg/day without significantly reducing the beneficial effect of the drug.

Retinoids

The side-effects of retinoids are characteristically those of hypervitaminosis A (Table 1.2).

Cheilitis – dry scaly lips – is an inevitable feature. Erythema of the face, often with some scaling, is also a virtually universal side-effect. Emollients, emollient oils for washing purposes and, if necessary, the use of 1% hydrocortisone ointment, usually relieve the problem. Occasionally stronger steroid ointments are required. Dryness of the nasal epithelia, and at times cracking, is again a characteristic feature of isotretinoin therapy but usually responds well to emollients. Conjunctivitis and blepharitis are seen frequently and if required the symptoms usually respond well to methyl cellulose eyedrops or polyvinyl alcohol eyedrops (Liquifilm).

A dermatitis may be seen on other areas of the body. The dermatitis

TABLE 1.2 Incidence of side-effects of patients taking isotretinoin

	Isotretinoin
Cheilitis	100%
Facial dermatitis	100%
Conjunctivitis	45%
Nasal dryness	77%
Alopecia	0%
Headaches	10%
Arthralgia	31%
Pyogenic granuloma	2%
DISH (diffuse interstitial skeletal hyperostosis)	<1%
Teratogenicity	100% risk
Elevated lipids (>normal)	19%
Elevated liver function (>normal)	12%

may simulate a primary irritant dermatitis on the hands; it may have a discoid appearance, or may even look like atopic eczema. The response to emollients, bath oils and weak steroid ointments is very satisfactory.

The drying of the skin with isotretinoin favours colonization of the skin with *Staphylococcus aureus* and frank impetigo or impetiginization of the dermatitis is not uncommon. Common sites of involvement are in association with the cheilitis and around the nose. An oral antibiotic such as erythromycin is often merited because of widespread colonization by the organisms.

Uncommon muco-cutaneous side-effects occur with a frequency of less than 2%. Fragility of the skin may be seen in athletic individuals. The onset of pyogenic granulomata if multiple can be quite disturbing to the acne patient but fortunately they respond well to treatment with either a potent topical corticosteroid ointment such as Dermovate NN (clobetasol, neomycin, nystatin), 1% silver nitrate in aqueous solution, or cautery and curettage. Such lesions are uncommon with etretinate.

The most important side-effect is that of teratogenicity[40]. There is a high incidence of cerebral, cardiac and aural defects and so if pregnancy does occur abortion is mandatory. Limited studies show no inter-reaction between the contraceptive pill and isotretinoin (0.5 mg/kg). Since the half life of isotretinoin is only 22 days, then contraception is required whilst on the drug and for 1 month afterwards.

Arthritis and vague aches and pains, especially in the legs and lower back are not uncommon but are usually mild and respond if needed to paracetamol. There could be a small but significant risk of the DISH syndrome (diffuse interstitial skeletal hyperostosis)[41]. This is a well recognized side effect of hypervitaminosis A in animals. DISH is also an age-dependent problem. It is recommended that an X-ray of the lumbar and cervical spine be taken in patients aged 35 or over and in any patient with a history of lower backache, prior to receiving the drug and at 4–6 monthly intervals. DISH is often asymptomatic but can sometimes produce limited and painful movement of the lumbar and cervical spine.

An unusual systemic side-effect ($<1\%$) is benign intracranial hypertension; this is the development of headache, loss of concentration, blurred vision and even papilloedema which can persist for 2 weeks after stopping therapy. This is easily diagnosed and patients taking the retinoids should not receive tetracycline as this drug also occasionally produces benign intracranial hypertension.

A whole range of other systemic side-effects have been reported – often single case reports. Other studies are necessary to substantiate such risks.

Isotretinoin will elevate bilirubin, alkaline phosphatase, liver enzymes, triglyceride and cholesterol (especially VHDL). The elevations are usually towards, or just beyond, the top limit of normal. The abnormalities are reversed within 2 weeks of stopping treatment. Rarely is it necessary to reduce or stop therapy because of these changes. The decision is more difficult in patients receiving etretinate because of its longer dose schedule. A risk of a triglyceride level 3–4 times normal is the development of pancreatitis; the significance of a temporarily raised VDRL and the potential risk of increased coronary vascular disease is uncertain.

FUTURE DEVELOPMENTS

One of the major obstacles preventing a better understanding of the aetiology of acne is the fact that acne is probably the most treatable of all chronic skin diseases and more attention is given to the less successfully treated diseases. Nevertheless we should still aim to find out more about the disease, the prime intention being to find a permanent cure. The fact that isotretinoin has such a long-term effect in obtaining remission in even the most severe of acne patients should give some clues to the molecular biologists.

Attention needs to be given to the end organ itself, the sebaceous gland, with probably less attention given to circulating hormones. One appreciates that any work on the pilosebaceous unit will almost certainly require an invasive technique – a biopsy. Recent evidence from our own department suggests that the sebaceous duct may also be androgen-controlled. We need to know much more about comedogenesis which is probably the least investigated aetiological aspect and such an investigation could give a clue to another important clinical feature of acne – which is why does it resolve spontaneously usually in the mid twenties? Evidence dictates that sebum excretion rate, as measured on the surface of the skin, is only slightly reduced in middle aged people and striking reductions in sebum excretion are only seen very late in life, well after acne has resolved.

The importance of bacteria, in particular *P. acnes*, has gone through phases of enthusiasm and lassitude. What is probably more relevant is a better understanding in the way that *P. acnes* colonizes the ducts and subsequently functions at that site both in health and disease.

Therapeutically there still exists a need for a topical drug which affects the two major important features of acne, that is the increased seborrhoea and comedogenesis. A successful topical anti-androgen would probably suffice this role but to date no successful topical anti-androgen is available and the reasons for this deficiency need to be determined. A topical retinoid as effective as 13-cis retinoic acid, but without its side-effects, particularly without the teratogenicity, would also fit the role of an ideal topical therapy.

It is unlikely that topical antimicrobial agents will influence more than inflammation and possibly to a lesser extent comedogenesis. Nevertheless since antimicrobial therapies have been the mainstay of acne therapy for many years they are likely to have an important role for some time. There is thus the need to produce non-sensitizing topical antimicrobial agents which act specifically against *P. acnes*, will not produce resistance and are concentrated to a very effective level in the pilosebaceous duct.

Since acne therapy has improved enormously in the last 15 years fewer patients should in the future develop scarring. Unfortunately some patients will scar and this emphasizes the important role of education. Doctors and patients must become aware of the better understanding of this disease and the way in which it should be managed.

REFERENCES

1. Kligman, A. M. and Mills, O. H. (1972). Acne cosmetica. *Arch. Dermatol.*, **106**, 843–50
2. Jowett, S. and Ryan, T. (1985). Skin disease and handicap: an analysis of the impact of skin conditions. *Soc. Sci. Med.*, **20**, 425–9
3. Marks, R. (1985). Acne – social impact and health education. *J. R. Soc. Med.* (Suppl.) **78**, 21–4
4. Gould, D. J. and Cunliffe, W. J. (1978). The long term treatment of acne vulgaris. *Clin. Exp. Dermatol.*, **3**, 249–52
5. Cunliffe, W. J., Forster, R. A., Greenwood, N. D., *et al.* (1973). Tetracycline and acne vulgaris: a clinical and laboratory investigation. *Br. Med. J.*, **4**, 332–5
6. Kirton, V. and Wilkinson, D. J. (1970). Benzoyl peroxide in acne. *Practitioner*, **204**, 683–6
7. Burke, B. M. and Cunliffe, W. J. (1984). The assessment of acne vulgaris – the Leeds technique. *Br. J. Dermatol.*, **111**, 83–92
8. Peachey, R. D. G. and Connor, B. L. (1971). Topical retinoic acid in the treatment of acne vulgaris. *Br. J. Dermatol.*, **85**, 462–6
9. Thomsen, R. J., Stranieri, A., Knutson, D. and Strauss, J. S. (1980). Topical clindamycin treatment of acne. *Arch. Dermatol.*, **116**, 1031–4
10. Pace, W. E. (1965). A benzoyl peroxide sulfur cream for acne vulgaris. *Can. Med. Assoc. J.*, **93**, 252–4
11. Cunliffe, W. J. and Shuster, S. (1969). Pathogenesis of acne. *Lancet*, **1**, 685–7
12. Fanta, D. and Jurecka, W. (1978). Autoradiographic investigation on benzoyl peroxide-treated skin. *Acta Dermatol. Venereol.*, **58**, 361–2
13. Cunliffe, W. J., Stainton, C. and Forster, R. A. (1983). Topical benzoyl peroxide increases the sebum excretion rate in patients with acne. *Br. J. Dermatol.*, **109**, 577–9
14. Mills, O. H. and Kligman, A. M. (1982). A human model for assaying comedolytic substances. *Br. J. Dermatol.*, **107**, 543–8
15. Cunliffe, W. J. and Holland, K. T. (1981). The effect of benzoyl peroxide on acne. *Acta Dermatol.*, **3**, 267–9
16. Stoughton, R. B. (1979). Topical antibiotics for acne vulgaris. *Arch. Dermatol.*, **115**, 486–9
17. Cunliffe, W. J., Burke, B. and Dodman, B. (1980). Chloramphenicol and benzoyl peroxide in acne. *Practitioner*, **224**, 952–4
18. Nazzaro-Porro, M., Passi, S., Picardo, M., Breathnach, A., Clayton, R. and Zina,

G. (1983). Beneficial effect of 15% azelaic acid cream on acne vulgaris. *Br. J. Dermatol.*, **109**, 45–8
19. Bladon, P. T., Burke, B. M., Cunliffe, W. J., Forster, R. A., Holland, K. T. and King, K. (1986). Topical azelaic acid and the treatment of acne: a clinical and laboratory comparison with oral tetracycline. *Br. J. Dermatol.*, **114**, 493–9
20. Mills, O. H. and Kligman, A. M. (1972). Is sulphur helpful or harmful in acne vulgaris? *Br. J. Dermatol.*, **86**, 620–7
21. Burton, J. L. (1979). Anti-androgen therapy in dermatology – a review. *Clin. Exp. Dermatol.*, **41**, 501–7
22. Baer, R. L., Leshaw, S. M. and Shalita, A. R. (1976). High dose tetracycline therapy in severe acne. *Arch. Dermatol.*, **112**, 479–81
23. Greenwood, R., Burke, B. and Cunliffe, W. J. (1986). Evaluation of a therapeutic strategy for the treatment of acne vulgaris with conventional therapy. *Br. J. Dermatol.*, **114**, 353–8
24. Pochi, P. E. and Strauss, J. S. (1973). Sebaceous gland suppression with ethinyl estradiol and diethylstilbestrol. *Arch. Dermatol.*, **108**, 210–4
25. Mugglestone, C. J. and Rhodes, E. L. (1982). The treatment of acne with an antiandrogen/oestrogen combination. *Clin. Exp. Dermatol.*, **7**, 593–8
26. Greenwood, R., Brummitt, L., Burke, B. and Cunliffe, W. J. (1986). Treatment of acne with either tetracycline, oestrogen/cyproterone acetate or combined therapy – a double blind laboratory and clinical study. *Br. J. Dermatol.* (In press)
27. Goodfellow, A., Alaghband-Zadeh, J., Carter, G., *et al.* (1984). Spironolactone improves acne vulgaris and reduces sebum excretion. *Br. J. Dermatol.*, **111**, 209–14
28. Strauss, J. A., Rapini, R. P., Shalita, A. R. *et al.* (1984). Isotretinoin therapy for acne. Results of a multicenter dose-response study. *J. Am. Acad. Dermatol.*, **10**, 490–6
29. Cunliffe, W. J., Jones, D. H., Pritlove, J. and Parkin, D. (1985). Long-term benefit of Isotretinoin in acne. *Retinoids: New Trends in Research and Therapy.* (Switzerland: S. Karger AG)
30. King, K., Jones, D. H., Daltrey, D. C. and Cunliffe, W. G. (1982). A double-blind study of the effects of 13-cis-retinoic acid on acne sebum excretion rate and microbial population. *Br. J. Dermatol.*, **107**, 583–90
31. Camisa, C., Elsenstat, B., Ragaz, A. and Wissman, G. (1982). The effects of retinoids on neutrophil functions *in vitro*. *J. Am. Acad. Dermatol.*, **6**, 620–9
32. Olsen, T. G. (1982). Therapy of acne. *Med. Clin. N. Am.*, **66**: pt. 4, 851–71
33. Peck, G. L., Olsen, T. G., Yoder, F. W., *et al.* (1979). Prolonged remissions in cystic and conglobate acne with 13-cis retinoic acid. *New Eng. J. Med.*, **62**, 191–201
34. Fulton, J. E., Marples, R., McGinley, K. and Leyden, J. J. (1968). Gram negative folliculitis in acne vulgaris. *Arch. Dermatol.*, **98**, 349–53
35. Klein, A. W. (1983). Implantation techniques for injectable collagen. *J. Am. Acad. Dermatol.*, **9**, 224–8
36. Goette, M. D. K. (1973). Liquid nitrogen in the treatment of acne vulgaris. *South. Med. J.*, **66**, 1131–2
37. Levine, R. M. and Rasmussen, J. E. (1983). Intralesional corticosteroids in the treatment of nodulocystic acne. *Arch. Dermatol.*, **119**, 480–1
38. Stuart, B. H. and Litt, I. F. (1978). Tetracycline-associated intracranial hypertension in an adolescent. A complication of systemic acne therapy. *J. Pediatr.*, **92**, 679–80

39. Liu, T.T.T. and May, N. (1985). Pigmentary changes due to long-term minocycline therapy. *Cutis*, **35**, 254–5
40. Chen, D.T. (1985). Human pregnancy experience with the retinoids. *Retinoids: New Trends in Research and Therapy*. (Switzerland: S. Karger AG)
41. McGuire, J., Milstone, L. and Lawson, J. (1985). Isotretinoin administration alters juvenile and adult bone. *Retinoids: New Trends in Research and Therapy*. (Switzerland: S. Karger AG)

2
LEG ULCERATION

D. J. BARKER

INTRODUCTION

Chronic leg ulcers are universally recognized as a major cause of discomfort and disability. They provide familiar problems for general practitioners, dermatologists, geriatricians and surgeons. Leg ulcers contribute substantially to the work of the community nursing services. Many ulcers can be healed but treatment is often difficult and always time-consuming. Slow progress inevitably leads to waning enthusiasm on the part of doctor, nurse and patient. It can justifiably be said that the chronic leg ulcer represents a disorder for which the physician is more likely to delegate than direct treatment.

How common is chronic ulceration of the leg? A recent postal survey in two Health Board areas in Scotland[1] identified 1477 patients with chronic ulcers in a population of one million. Extrapolating from their findings the authors suggest that there may be 400 000 people in the UK with active or recently healed ulcers. A survey in an English Health District[2] located 337 leg ulcer patients in a population of 198 000. Both studies indicated that women with leg ulcers outnumber men by 2:1, and that the great majority of patients are managed entirely within the community. From this it naturally follows that a new drug, dressing, or treatment technique, appropriate only to a specialist hospital department may not make a significant impact on the overall problem. It is the frequent, and entirely justified, complaint of community nurses in the UK that valuable new dressings available to hospitals are not prescribable by general practitioners.

Clearly the recognition of a leg ulcer is not in itself a sufficient diagnosis. Ulceration always indicates some underlying disease, frequently circulatory. Treatment must be directed towards healing the ulcer, but also the problem that permitted ulceration to occur should be corrected. In reality both these objectives are pursued simultaneously with the second proving difficult, or sometimes impossible, to attain.

A vast number of drugs, bandages, dressings and topical applications are marketed for the treatment of leg ulcers. Many are useless and some are positively harmful. Older agents, such as honey, were employed by the ancient Greeks and have thus been in continuous use for 2000 years. The individual assessment of these products is bedevilled by the fact that few seem to have been subjected to good controlled clinical trials. The results of the trials that are published often appear contradictory. In fairness one must say that the complexity of the events that lead to ulceration, and our ignorance of the healing processes, do make trials difficult to organize and interpret. After a long period of apparent disinterest the pharmaceutical industry has recently produced many exciting new dressing materials. Unfortunately the sheer numbers of these new products has further obscured an already confusing situation. It will take wisdom indeed to separate the gold from the dross. It is hardly necessary to add that materials which appear highly effective when applied to standard wounds of laboratory pigs may perform less well when used to treat chronic multifactorial ulcers in elderly humans.

Recently it has been the surgeons and pharmacologists who have contributed most to our understanding of the patho-physiology of ulceration. However dermatologists have a very definite role in elucidating the rarer causes of ulcer formation, and in practice direct a great deal of treatment. Dermatologists also deserve credit for recognizing the damage caused by sensitizers in many widely used local preparations. As things stand however there can be no doubt that many ulcer patients are poorly managed. There is little uniformity in treatment practices, and communication between hospital-based and community services is often poor. There is little formal evaluation of treatment techniques in either group. This situation should be improved if at all possible.

In this chapter I shall describe the causes of ulceration, and follow this with a discussion of wound healing together with the general principles of treatment. I shall then deal with the specific management of ulcer-promoting conditions, and in particular with venous disease of the legs.

DIAGNOSIS AND ASSESSMENT OF LEG ULCERS

The presence of a section devoted to diagnosis, in a chapter concerned with treatment needs explanation, but not apology. Often difficulties with ulcer management originate from incorrect diagnosis or incomplete initial assessment. Although the majority of leg ulcers are of vascular origin some are not and, for these, specific and often rapidly effective treatment may exist. Even in individuals with unquestionable vascular ulceration it is essential to determine the relative contributions of venous and arterial disease since this information profoundly affects subsequent management.

Venous ulcers

In the UK some 80% of leg ulcers are venous in origin. In many instances minor trauma or infection finally precipitates ulceration in skin damaged by long-standing venous disease. Venous ulcers are superficial, irregular and relatively painless. They commonly involve the 'gaiter' area of the lower leg (Figure 2.1). The two most important physical signs pointing to the venous origin of an ulcer are haemosiderin pigmentation and a flare of dilated venules below the medial malleolus. Varicose superficial veins, oedema, induration and atrophie blanche (Figure 2.2) are frequently, but not invariably, present. The actual ulcer surface consists of fibro-vascular granulation tissue with a variable admixture of fibrinous slough. The initial assessment of a venous ulcer should include a careful recording of its size and shape. In the absence of spreading infection the culture of a wound swab is unlikely to provide valuable information. In addition to urinalysis and routine blood investigations an early patch test should be considered. Venous ulcer patients are particularly prone to the development of a medicament dermatitis. One study[3] showed that 81% of subjects tested

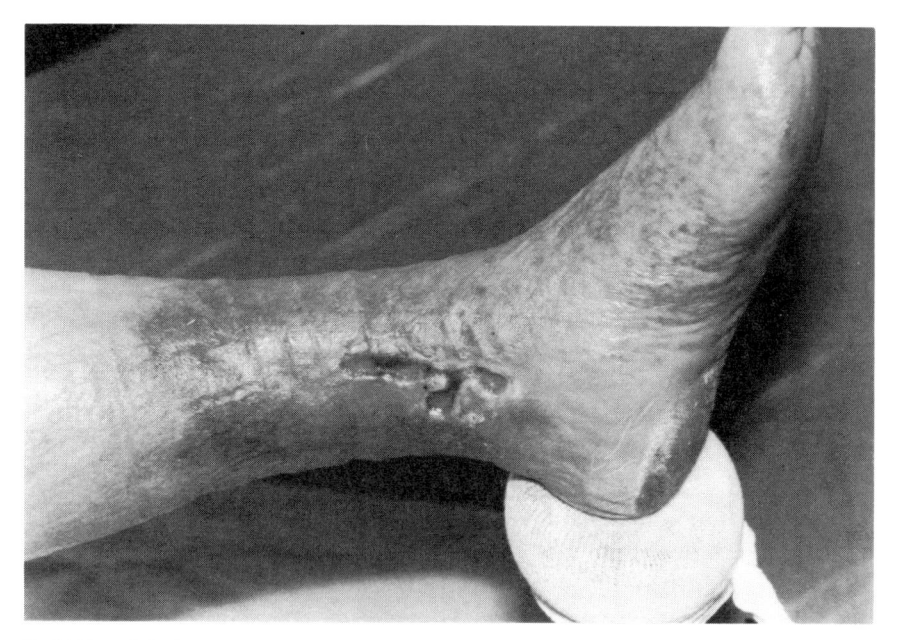

FIGURE 2.1 Typical venous leg ulcer

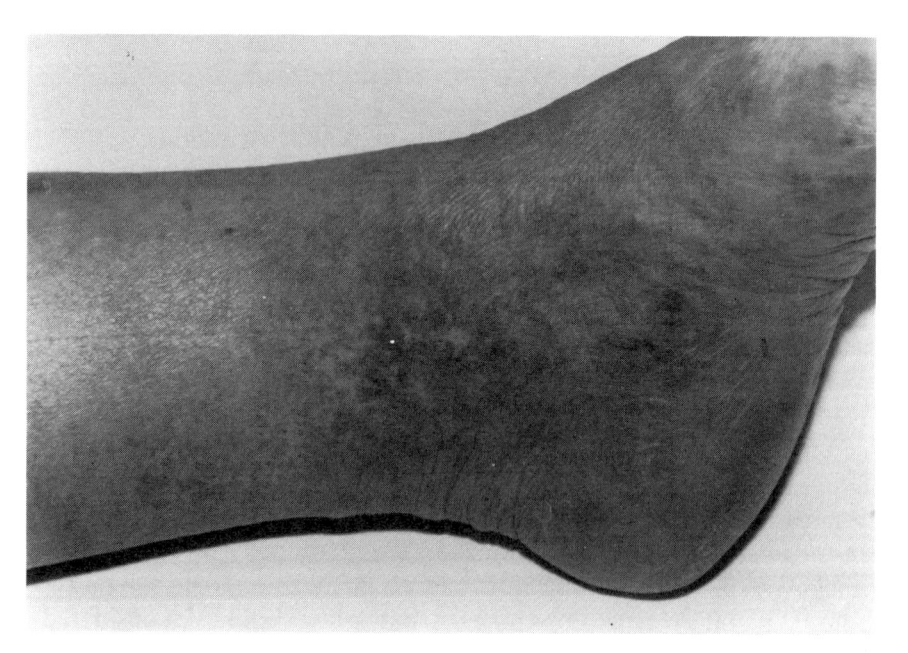

FIGURE 2.2 Atrophie blanche

had one or more positive patch test reactions. Assessment of the affected limb by venography may be valuable if surgery is being planned.

Arterial ulceration

Arterial, or ischaemic, ulceration is painful; typically the discomfort is worst at night when the limb is elevated in bed. The ulcers are 'punched-out', deep and contain thick, necrotic slough. There is loss of deep fascia and tendons or muscles may be exposed. Any part of the leg may be involved but the toes, dorsum of the foot, heel, or anterior tibial area are common locations. The skin of the ischaemic foot is shiny, hairless, pink and very susceptible to pressure-induced necrosis. Such patients may develop small but extremely painful ulcers over the malleoli or the heads of the first and fifth metatarsals; all these sites are subject to pressure from footwear. The peripheral pulses will very often not be palpable in patients suffering from peripheral vascular disease. It is unwise however to rely on this physical sign particularly in the presence of oedema. The ankle systolic pressure can be measured directly using a Doppler ultra-sound technique[4]. An index can then be calculated if the ankle pressure is divided by the brachial pressure. Normal individuals will have an index of 1 or greater. An arterial pressure index below 0.7 would certainly justify arteriographic investigation and surgical referral. Many presumed venous ulcers, particularly in the elderly, have an arterial element and are more correctly described as 'mixed' ulcers. This situation should be suspected if an apparently venous ulcer in an elderly patient proves unexpectedly painful or slow to heal. Under such circumstances the estimation of an arterial pressure index is essential.

Leg ulcers in diabetics

The factors responsible for the development of diabetic ulcers are neuropathy, ischaemia and infection. Chronic plantar ulceration is commonly the result of diabetic peripheral nerve damage although other neuropathies (e.g. alcoholic, leprotic and hereditary) can produce an identical pattern. The ulceration is the consequence of repeated chronic trauma in patients whose impaired sensory innervation deprives them of 'pain protection'. Infected sinuses may form over the weight-bearing metatarsal heads. Ischaemic ulcers may form on the toes and are frequently complicated by infection. Altogether the swollen, infected and ischaemic diabetic foot is a most testing clinical challenge. A rarer cause of leg ulceration in diabetics is an ulcerated area of necrobiosis lipoidica, usually on the pre-tibial area.

Other causes of ulceration

Dermal atrophy occurs with advancing age. The skin becomes inelastic and parchment-thin. Trauma easily leads to pre-tibial tears, or venous rupture with the formation of large subcutaneous haematomas. Early surgical removal of devitalized tissue with split-skin grafting is recommended in such circumstances since attempts at conservative treatment usually result in long-lasting ulceration. Sadly an all too common source of trauma to elderly legs is pressure from over-tight bandages.

The significance of bacteria present on chronic leg ulcers has been exaggerated in the past but unquestionably severe superficial infection with the haemolytic streptococcus or *Staphylococcus aureus* can produce a true infective ulcer which will respond to antibiotic treatment alone. In the UK other infective causes of leg ulceration, such as tuberculosis and tertiary syphilis, are now most uncommon. This situation is not, of course, true world-wide. I have neither the space nor the experience to deal adequately with the causes of leg ulceration encountered in the tropical and sub-tropical areas of the world. Several conditions must at least be mentioned. Subcutaneous fungal infections such as chromoblastomycosis and sporotrichosis frequently affect the foot producing ulceration. The 'tropical ulcer' is often endemic in these areas; this is an acute ulcer, usually of the lower leg, which is associated with malnutrition and is caused by infection with bacteria such as *Borrelia vincenti*. Leprosy and the results of the neuropathy

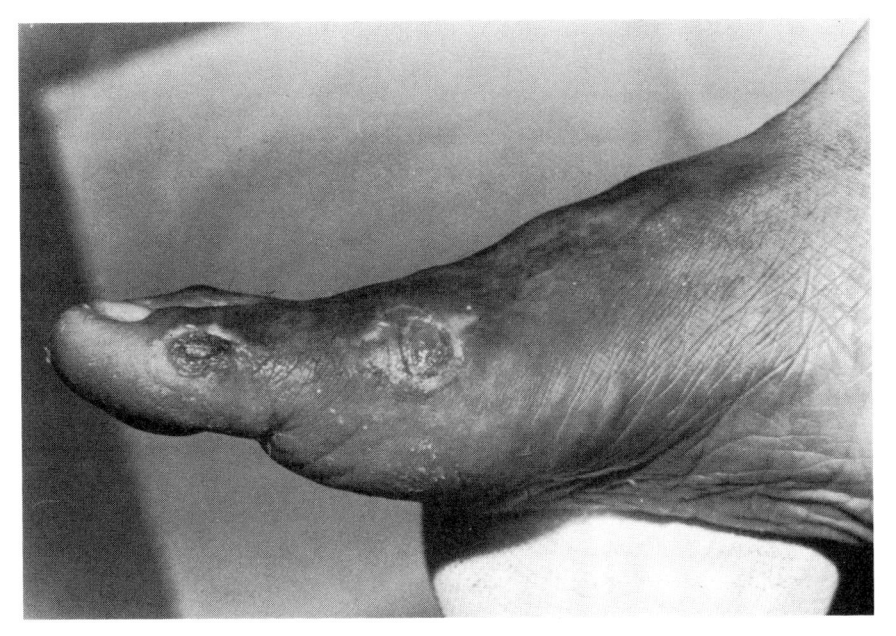

FIGURE 2.3 Neuropathic ulcers (leprosy)

that it produces are familiar problems (Figure 2.3).

Squamous cell carcinomas have long been recognized as complicating long-standing leg ulceration of several types. It has recently become clear that basal cell carcinomas also have this propensity[5]. This situation is almost certainly under-reported and must be considered if any ulcer suddenly enlarges, develops a raised edge or unexpectedly fails to respond to treatment. Malignant melanomas may occur on the sole and if poorly melanized may resemble an ulcerated mass of granulation tissue. Biopsy is mandatory if the true nature of an ulcer is in doubt. It is wise to biopsy several sites in the centre and periphery of such an ulcer.

Leg ulcers are a well-recognized complication of homozygous sickle-cell disease, thalassaemia and hereditary spherocytosis[6]. Like venous ulcers they predominantly affect the 'gaiter' area and may be precipitated by trauma. Indeed it seems likely that venous factors play a part in determining the site of ulceration. In these diseases the erythrocytes are unduly rigid showing reduced deformability. Sickle cell disease is associated with increased blood viscosity. Both these factors would accentuate hypoxia in an area with poor arterial circulation.

Pyoderma gangrenosum is a rapidly developing ulcerative and inflammatory dermatosis. It is often associated with inflammatory bowel disease, rheumatoid arthritis or the myelo-proliferative disorders although it may occur in isolation. The diagnosis of pyoderma gangrenosum should be considered whenever a rapidly expanding leg ulcer fails to respond to conventional treatment. Classically there will be a central necrotic ulcer surrounded by a swollen cyanotic margin and, external to that, an erythematous flare. There are other causes of leg ulceration in rheumatoid disease. Both small dermal infarcts and larger, more penetrating, ulcers may form. The principal cause is a vasculitis involving small and medium sized vessels. In arthritic patients the treatment of the ulcers is often complicated by immobility, and the consequences of cortico-steroid therapy. Other types of lower limb vasculitis may produce ulceration. These include systemic lupus erythematosus, hydralazine-induced lupus erythematosus, systemic sclerosis, and acute necrotizing vasculitis.

Finally it must be emphasized that not all leg ulcers are organic in origin. Dermatitis artefacta must be considered if the ulcer is linear or geometrical in shape; there may be superficial necrosis. Typically, artefactual ulcers heal with occlusive dressing but the long-term management of such patients can be most difficult (Figure 2.4).

WOUND HEALING AND THE LOCAL TREATMENT OF ULCERS

Chronic cutaneous ulceration represents loss of the epidermis with portions of dermal and subcutaneous tissues. Krull[7] has emphasized that except for pressure sores chronic skin ulceration is virtually synonymous with leg ulcers, so frequently are they found on the lower limb distal to the knee. Assuming that we can correct or at least ameliorate the underlying disease process, how will the ulcer heal? Full-thickness wound healing is a complex process. Naturally much of the investigative work has been performed on standard, reproducible wounds rather than on the confused battlefield of destruction, regeneration and infection that is represented by an actual leg ulcer.

Ultimately healing of an ulcer will occur by means of granulation

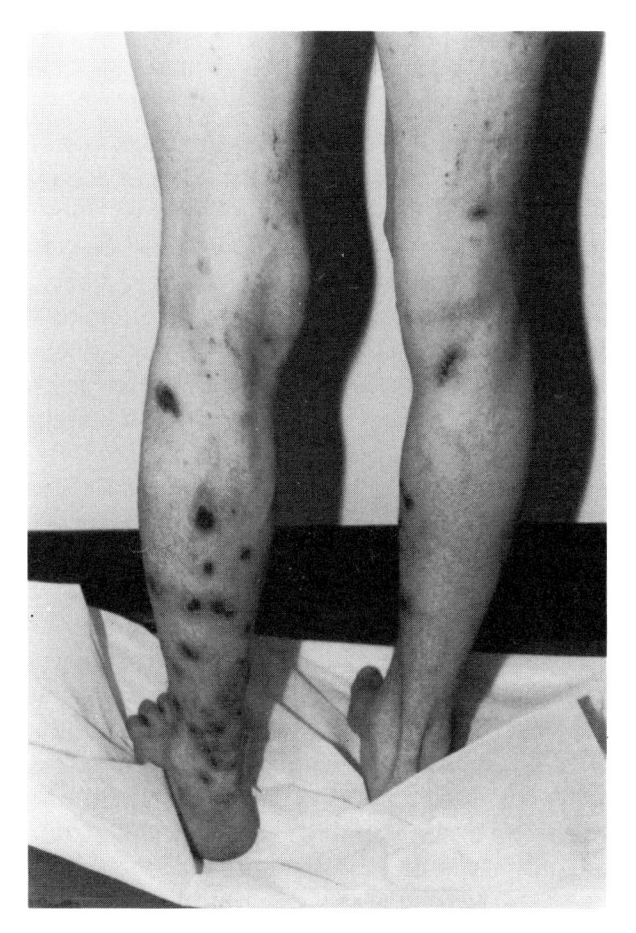

FIGURE 2.4 Artefactual leg ulcers

tissue formation resulting in wound contraction. Later the granulation tissue is re-epithelialized from the periphery, and from residual epidermal remnants in the ulcer itself. Later still there will be dermal remodelling in the old ulcer base. How can a microenvironment be created to enhance these healing processes? A dry environment leads to scab formation which impedes epithelial cell migration; occlusion of some type will create a moist wound with an increased rate of re-epithelialization[8]. A moist wound also hastens the appearance of dermal fibroblasts. The role of oxygen is more complicated and this important subject has been reviewed recently by Silver[9]. Oxygen is necessary for effective wound healing but its beneficial effects are more obvious on epithelial than connective tissues. Macrophages have a vital function in ulcer healing since they produce an angiogenic factor thus stimulating new vessel growth. The release of angiogenic factor is enhanced by hypoxic conditions and this may offset the other disadvantages of hypoxia. In fact there seems to be agreement[9, 10] that the PO_2 of fluid bathing chronic infected leg ulcers is very low even if oxygen-permeable dressings are employed. The implication of this work is that normal regeneration of this type of full-thickness wound takes place in a low oxygen environment with the oxygen required for the process originating in the local blood supply and not by diffusion from the ulcer surface.

Despite the potential benefits, the use of occlusive ulcer dressings has been criticized on the grounds that they will promote infection. Although bacteria are plentiful on the surface of an ulcer, which indeed may harbour several species, it is doubtful if they are often of any real clinical significance. In one study[11] it was demonstrated that while the healing of venous ulcers did indeed correlate with declining bacterial counts these counts were not favourably affected by an antiseptic. Eriksson[12] found that patients kept their ulcer's original bacterial flora irrespective of the type and effects of treatment. In addition there were no differences in bacterial findings between ulcers clinically judged to be 'clean' and those considered 'dirty'. The evaluation of bacterial species present on an ulcer provides the laboratory with a great deal of work to very little purpose. The situation is quite different if there is evidence of spreading cellulitis originating from the ulcer. Under these circumstances culture of the organism responsible and the determination of antibiotic sensitivities may be valuable. The situation is similar if a split-skin graft is contemplated. The presence of *Staphylococcus aureus* or *Pseudomonas pyocyanea* (*aeruginosa*) is associated with diminished graft survival.

The materials applied to wounds can be divided rather arbitrarily into three classes.

(1) Debriding and cleansing agents;
(2) Absorbent materials;
(3) Occlusive dressings.

This complex situation has been reviewed recently[13]. The ideal material would be cheap, painless and non-sensitizing. It would be non-adherent and on removal would leave no residue to be incorporated into the healing wound. Finally an optimum environment for wound healing would be created. In practice these requirements are difficult to attain.

Debriding and cleansing agents

Gentle debridement of an ulcer with removal of slough and necrotic debris is an essential preliminary to the formation of healthy granulation tissue. The cautious use of scalpel, scissors and forceps is unbeatable for this purpose. Specific debriding topical preparations such as streptokinase/streptodornase (Varidase) and mixtures of malic, benzoic and salicylic acids (Aserbine; Malatex) have been in use for many years. I have not found them to be very effective. Certainly the adequate debridement of an ulcer with reduction of oedema is of far greater importance to its subsequent healing than the application of antimicrobial agents to the surface. There is no justification whatever for the use of topical antibiotics, such as neomycin or gentamicin. It is doubtful if these substances aid healing in any way. Besides their doubtful efficacy the use of such antibiotics fosters the emergence of resistant strains of bacteria, and risks sensitization of the patient. Preparations containing weaker sensitizers like lanolin, chlorocresol or preservatives of the parabens group may also lead to the development of a medicament dermatitis, a complication to which patients with leg ulcers are particularly prone[3]. Ulcer therapists must be vigilant and also remember that sometimes an obvious acute dermatitis does not occur; in these cases the ulcer will simply fail to heal until the sensitizer is recognized and removed.

Eusol is a solution of calcium hypochlorite and boric acid. It is used for cleansing ulcers and as a general purpose antiseptic. Sodium hypochlorite has similar properties. Cetrimide (a mixture of quaternary ammonium compounds), chlorhexidine gluconate and povidone iodine have all been employed for ulcer cleaning. Use of any antiseptic seems based on a fundamental misconception concerning the importance of bacterial infection; furthermore their toxicity has been underestimated in the past. Many antiseptics have been tested for their effects on granulation tissue using a rabbit's ear chamber model[14]. All the antiseptics tested caused some adverse effects, and the hypochlorites were found to be extremely damaging to the capillary circulation and the process of repair.

Rosaniline dyes are cheap and seldom sensitize. A $\frac{1}{2}$% aqueous solution of crystal (gentian) violet has been painted on leg ulcers for decades. Brilliant green has acquired a new lease of life following its incorporation with lactic acid into a gel for leg ulcer application (Variclene). For placebo value the rosaniline dyes probably have no equal but efficacy has never been clearly demonstrated and their use is declining. Oxidizing agents such as hydrogen peroxide, zinc peroxide and 20% benzoyl peroxide have been widely used although pain may be a problem. Hioxyl is a 1.5% stabilized hydrogen peroxide cream. It is certainly convenient, well-tolerated and non-sensitizing but its value as a healing agent remains unproven.

Absorbent materials

All ulcer therapists are familiar with the problem of dressing adherence. If the dressing sticks then its removal will damage the fragile regenerating epidermis. Traditionally a piece of plain paraffin gauze is cut to size and placed on the ulcer followed by a pad of sterile gauze material. This pad serves to soak up exudate and perhaps to distribute more evenly the pressure of any overlying bandage. The use of antibiotic-impregnated paraffin gauze (e.g. Sofratulle; Fucidin Tulle) seems irrational for the reasons already stated. Even plain paraffin gauze has the disadvantage of leaving materials behind which could become incorporated into the wound. One alternative is a square of activated charcoal cloth (Actisorb). This is heat-sealed, non-adherent and highly absorbent. It is particularly valuable in profusely exudative and maloderous ulcers.

The most familiar of the newer topical preparations are the absorbent carbohydrate polymers. These are formulated into powders consisting of inert, hydrophilic, spherical microbeads. When applied to ulcers these products absorb exudate and remove particulate material. The first carbohydrate polymer to be marketed in the UK was dextranomer (Debrisan). Another system, cadexomer iodine (Iodosorb), is a modified starch polymer that releases iodine as it absorbs. A starch co-polymer hydrogel (Scherisorb) is also available. Naturally the application techniques of these products are not identical. In general however the ulcer is cleaned and then covered with a layer of polymer 3–4 mm thick. A dry dressing is applied next. When the dressing is changed the old material should be washed off with a stream of water or saline, this causing minimal damage to the regenerating epidermis. Once the polymer becomes saturated with exudate the benefits resulting from its presence cease. Ideally the powder should be replaced before saturation occurs and in practice once or twice daily treatment is necessary. A great deal of literature has been devoted to the subject of polymers. Despite this it is not possible to state unequivocally whether polymers really aid ulcer healing; or whether one polymer is better than any other. Some investigators have obtained good results with dextranomer or cadexomer iodine[15], others have found neither helpful[16]. In evaluating these products one should not ignore their relatively high cost. They are not really suitable for dry ulcers. If they are used it is important to follow the manufacturer's recommended techniques closely and to record ulcer size so that some objective evidence of healing, or lack of healing, is obtained.

Alginates are salts of alginic acid, derived from various brown seaweeds. Their chemical structure is that of a complex polyuronide. Calcium alginate is insoluble but in the presence of excess sodium ions a soluble sodium alginate gel is formed. Calcium alginate fibre squares are marketed as Sorbsan and Kaltostat. If squares are placed over an ulcer, exudate and tissue fluid are absorbed to form a hydrophilic gel over the surface of the wound. This provides a moist environment suitable for wound healing. Calcium alginate is biodegradable and is easily removed by washing away with saline, this process being commendably atraumatic to the healing ulcer. Calcium alginate has no directly anti-microbial properties although this probably presents no great loss. The product is easy to apply and non-sensitizing; as yet however no formal trials have been published evaluating its clinical performance in the treatment of leg ulcers.

Geliperm is an inert polyacrylamide/agar hydrogel. It is formulated as a transparent moist gel sheet which is non-adhering, gas permeable and adopts the contours of the wound to which it is applied. It combines a high moisture content which should encourage epidermal cell migration, with a high absorptive capacity. The ulcer can, of course, be inspected through the sheet. If required, antiseptics can be incorporated into the matrix of the gel by soaking it in the chosen antiseptic solution prior to application. Geliperm is expensive but should certainly be considered for patients who find conventional dressings intolerably painful. Geliperm is also available in a granulated form the use of which resembles that of the polymer absorbent materials described above.

Occlusive dressings

Synthetic pliable occlusive skin dressings have recently become very popular in the UK. My only personal experience so far has been with Granuflex although several other similar products will shortly become available. Granuflex has been described as an occlusive hydrocolloid and is a sheet consisting of an adhesive inner face, and an outer surface of an impervious foam. The hydrocolloid contains gelatin, pectin and carboxymethylcellulose. Once the dressing is applied the exudate from the ulcer is absorbed to produce a gel between the ulcer surface and the dressing. This gel has a penetrating and unpleasant odour but fortunately this is only a problem if the dressing leaks. Dressing removal is easy, painless and atraumatic with surplus gel being washed away with water. The dressing should be changed twice weekly unless leakage occurs. The sheets are non-sensitizing and can be worn under a support dressing or an elastic stocking. Following the initial application of the dressing a degree of 'auto-debridement' occurs with a paradoxical enlargement of the ulcer. One possible disadvantage in the use of occlusive dressings of this type is that bacterial proliferation might be encouraged. This problem has been studied with six semi-permeable occlusive dressings available in the USA[17]. The authors induced standard wounds in volunteers and then ascertained whether there were any differences in the rates of healing dependant on which dressing was selected. Similar wounds were investigated after they had been inoculated with four different pathogenic bacteria. It was shown that there were no significant differences in the rates of healing and that none of the dressings had the capacity to stave off infection once a pathogen was introduced. This situation may not of course be entirely analogous with that of a chronic leg ulcer. Certainly severe infection has not been a major problem during my use of occlusive dressing materials.

In addition to synthetic substances a number of biological dressings have been devised. They are not helpful in inflamed or necrotic ulcers but appear to hasten healing and diminish pain when a healthy bed of granulation tissue is established. Skin grafts were an early biological dressing and are still popular. Many dermatologists would favour pinch-grafting rather than formal split-skin grafting. Admittedly the final cosmetic result is poorer but the technique is easy, the percentage of 'take' is high, and the regenerated ulcer surface thicker. Grafting can dramatically shorten ulcer healing time and has been successfully applied both to hospital in-patients and on an out-patient basis. Experimentally human amnion applied to leg ulcers has enhanced healing but in practice porcine dermis is the most feasible biological dressing at present. Lyophilized freeze-dried dermis (Corethium-2) is reconstituted in physiological saline, cut to shape, and applied to the wound under conventional dressings. The procedure should be repeated once or twice weekly; the area of porcine dermis required declines as healing takes place.

THE AETIOLOGY AND TREATMENT OF VENOUS ULCERS

The link between venous disease and leg ulceration has been recognized for centuries. It is only in the last few years that a convincing explanation of the association has emerged. The fundamental cause of the ulceration is sustained venous hypertension in the veins around the ankle. The questions that we must answer are firstly how does venous hypertension develop, and secondly, how do ulcers develop as a consequence? The work of several investigative vascular surgeons has placed us in a good position to explain both problems, and as a result we can begin to plan treatment on a more rational basis.

The veins of the leg can be considered as two systems. The superficial (long saphenous and short saphenous veins with their tributaries) and the deep veins. The deep system is represented by the muscular sinuses and the tibial and peroneal veins which enter the popliteal vein, ultimately forming the femoral vein. The superficial and deep systems unite at the sapheno-femoral junction but are also linked by perforating veins, so called because they perforate or penetrate the deep fascia. The number of perforating veins is variable but may be 50–100. Some are highly inconstant but others are more consistently present, these including three adjacent to the medial malleolus and one adjacent to the lateral malleolus. Perforating veins contain valves which permit blood to flow only from the low pressure superficial system to the high pressure deep system of veins. During exercise skeletal muscle compression pushes the blood out of the soleal sinuses and deep veins onward into the popliteal vein and ultimately the inferior vena cava. When the muscles relax reflux of blood from the deep veins is prevented by valves. Because of the consequent low pressure blood can now flow from the superficial system through the perforators into the deep veins. As a result the pressure in the superficial veins also falls. The effects of these mechanisms are quite considerable; on quiet standing the venous pressure at the ankle is 85–90 mmHg, on exercise this pressure drops to 30 mmHg.

It has been appreciated for many years that venous ulcers could occur in the absence of varicose veins. Despite a common misconception the idea that ulceration results from the presence of 'static' blood lying in dilated leg veins is now discredited. If there were significant stasis of venous blood in an affected limb then the oxygenation of the femoral venous blood would be expected to fall. In fact patients with unilateral varicose veins have a higher femoral vein blood oxygen content on the affected side than on the control side. Such a limb also shows an increased blood flow. These findings lead to the postulation that arterio-venous communications, present in normal individuals, opened up in response to venous obstruction, thus this promoting the development of ulceration by reducing skin blood flow. Attempts to demonstrate the presence of these fistulae have however failed to show consistent evidence of their existence.

It is now believed that if perforating vein valves are damaged, then during exercise the high pressures generated in the deep veins can be directly transmitted through the now incompetent perforators into the superficial system. In short there is an explosive injection of high pressure blood occurring at regular intervals. Using ultrasound flow detectors it is actually possible to demonstrate reversed blood through incompetent perforating veins during muscle contraction.

It was initially assumed that damage to the deep and perforating veins followed one or more episodes of deep venous thrombosis. Indeed a lower limb manifesting varicose veins, oedema, pigmentation and liposclerosis began to be described as a 'post-phlebitic leg'. Browse and colleagues[18] studied 130 legs belonging to 67 patients 5–10 years after a phlebographically proven deep venous thrombosis. The study did not include an ideal control group (patients who were clinically and venographically normal) but their results were extremely interesting. They found that only 20% of legs previously affected by a severe thrombosis had marked post-phlebitic symptoms when re-examined, whilst 2% of legs which had shown no evidence of a thrombosis had later developed such symptoms. The overall conclusion drawn from this work was that the development of 'post-phlebitic syndrome' can be unpredictable. It seems clear that factors other than thrombosis can damage the valves of perforating veins. If the calf muscle pump mechanism fails transmitted pressure alone may damage the valves. In 'pure' sapheno-femoral incompetence the whole saphenous vein system and its tributaries can become varicose. Competent ankle perforators can protect the ankle region from damage for many years but ultimately the valves may fail for hydrostatic reasons. In other instances it has been suggested that intrinsic disease of the valve, or vein wall, is responsible for valvular incompetence. Whatever the mechanism it is puzzling that venous ulceration so selectively affects the region of the ankle. The perforating veins in this area (between the tibia and soleus muscle) are large, short, unsupported by muscle, and contain only one valve. For these reasons they may be particularly susceptible to damage. This region is also poorly vascularized by small perforating arteries when compared with the adjacent heel and calf.

The elucidation of the link between venous hypertension and ulceration is clearly of critical importance. Burnand and Browse[19] noted that venous hypertension lead to an increase in the size of the dermal capillary bed. The degree of this change can be correlated with elevation of pedal venous pressure after exercise. They made the further suggestion that the high pressure transmitted to the capillary circulation widens endothelial pores and this in turn permits fibrinogen (but not larger molecules such as albumin) to escape into the interstitial fluid. Here fibrin is formed and deposited around the capillaries where it can be detected histologically. It has been suggested that the presence of this pericapillary fibrin impairs the diffusion of oxygen. As a result the skin and subcutaneous tissue become hypoxic, and are therefore more susceptible to ulceration. *In vitro* fibrin sheets reduce the diffusion of oxygen as compared to that of carbon dioxide. Strong confirmation of this theory would be provided by the demonstration, *in vivo*, of reduced oxygen diffusion into the skin in individuals suffering from venous disease. Regional oxygen utilization and blood flow has been studied using positron emission tomographic scanning after the continuous inhalation of oxygen-15[20]. The results showed that lipodermatosclerotic tissue and ulcer bearing skin had a very high blood flow, reflecting the proliferation of capillaries in these tissues, but a greatly reduced oxygen extraction. The technique described is complex but the results achieved do seem to support the hypothesis of the pericapillary fibrin cuff.

If fibrin deposition is ultimately responsible for the skin changes associated with venous disease then clearly its removal by the stimulation of fibrinolysis might prove profitable. There is evidence that both blood and tissue fibrinolytic activity are significantly depressed in patients suffering from venous disease[19] although it is not established if this is a primary or secondary change. Unremoved the fibrin deposited in the tissues would ultimately be replaced, irreversibly, by scar tissue.

The pericapillary fibrin diffusion block theory has not yet reached the stage of universal acceptance but it seems to explain all the observed phenomena. There may however be systemic factors of relevance unconnected with fibrin deposition. Goodfield[21] has shown an increase in platelet number and volume in patients with venous eczema and ulcers when compared with normal controls. These platelet parameters do not change following the healing of the ulcers, and thus they may be a primary feature of venous disease.

Virtually all pure venous ulcers in mobile patients can be induced to heal if oedema is controlled and venous drainage improved. These objectives can be achieved by prolonged bed-rest, but for practical reasons ambulatory treatment is used in the majority of cases. The achievement of graduated compression of the leg is gaining acceptance as the single most important aspect of conservative management, indeed it is the one aspect of venous ulcer treatment of which all authorities approve. It is not however entirely without risk. Any form of external compression is forbidden in ischaemic ulceration since this can further reduce an already compromised circulation. Failure to accurately assess the cause of ulceration can therefore have disastrous consequences. For patients with genuinely 'mixed' ulcers it can be a matter of very nice judgement whether there is more to be lost or gained by providing support. External compression retards the development of oedema and reverses the haemodynamic consequences of muscle pump failure and perforator incompetence. The precise degree of compression required to give optimal benefit to patients with venous disease is uncertain. Values of 30–40 mmHg at the ankle graduating to 20 mmHg compression at the knee are often quoted. This degree of external support can be provided in either of two ways; compression bandaging or support stockings. Employed correctly both techniques can be successful. I should like to discuss them individually before contrasting their merits.

Compression bandaging is still widely used in the UK. There are considerable variations in the methods of application and the materials used. I must point out that correct technique can only be learned under direct supervision by an experienced practitioner. Once the ulcer has been cleaned the first step is the application of a paste bandage (Figure 2.5). A paste bandage consists of a bleached cotton strip 7.5 cm wide and 6 m in length. The cotton is impregnated with zinc oxide, starch and glycerine. A preservative, in the UK normally of the parabens group, is incorporated and this occasionally causes sensitivity problems. The paste bandage holds any dressings in place and acts as a buffer between the overlying compression bandage and the skin. There is evidence that the presence of a paste bandage enhances and prolongs the ability of the compression bandage to maintain its support[22]. Strips of the paste bandage are applied in an annular pattern from the base of the toes to the tibial tuberosity. It is important to obtain a smooth finish without any folds or tucks that could result in pressure necrosis of the underlying skin. There are a great many paste bandages available; in the UK Zincaband or Viscopaste PB7 would be suitable.

The final stage in the procedure is the application of a compression bandage (Figure 2.6). Several of these are in common use; examples are 7.5 cm adhesive zinc oxide strapping (Poroplast) and the elastic diachylon bandage (Lestreflex) which uses a lead oleate and resin

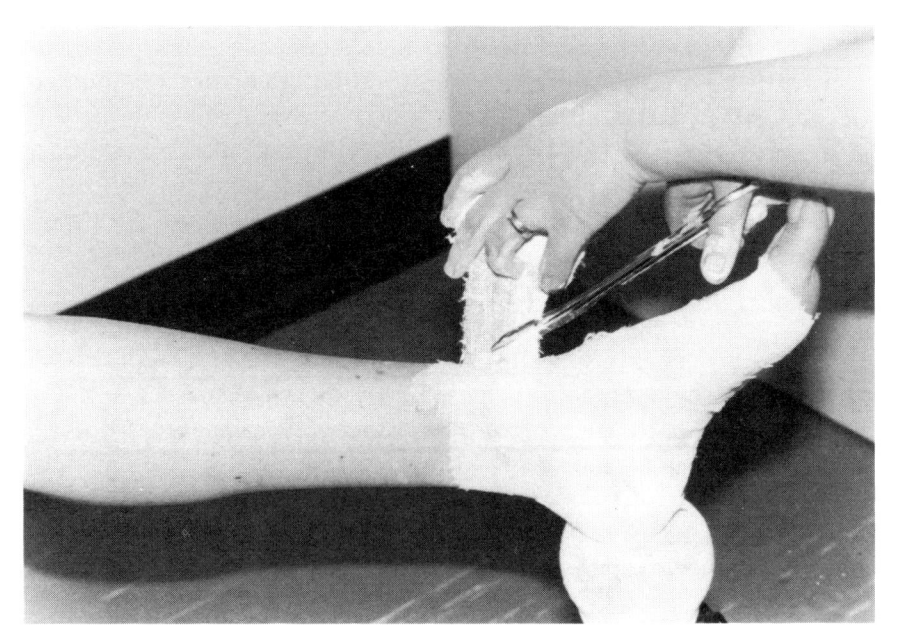

FIGURE 2.5 Application of a paste bandage

adhesive. Lestreflex is flesh-coloured and easy to apply but requires warming before use. An elastic cohesive bandage (Secure Forte) is a useful new addition. It consists of a cotton, viscose, polyurethane mix and has the useful property of sticking only to itself. The bandage is comfortable to wear and provides adequate support for a weekly dressing. It can even be washed once or twice without losing too much elasticity. The capacity of any bandage to exert compression is partly determined by the materials from which it is made, and partly by the tension generated during application. When applying the bandage it is important to maintain an even tension or 'pull'. Naturally this takes a good deal of experience. Pressure measurements have actually been made under applied bandages using a suitable sensor[22]. Results show that a single practised operator is reasonably consistent in performance and can judge the degree of tension required with surprising accuracy.

Before applying the bandage the patient should be asked to hold the foot at a 90 degree angle to the leg. A 25 cm strip of bandage should be pulled out and wrapped round the heel. Next a turn should be taken round the base of the toes. After completing the cover of the

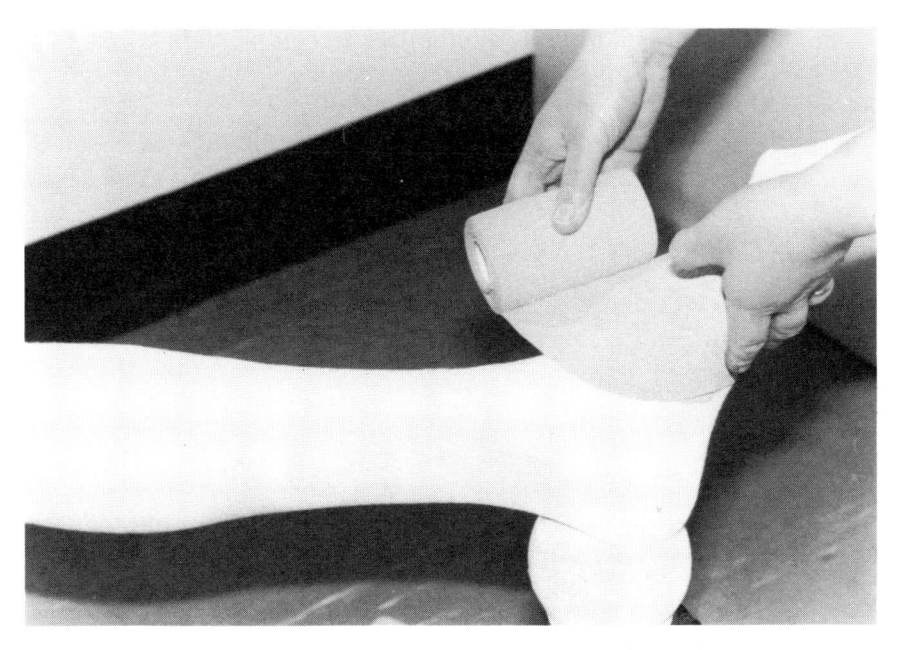

FIGURE 2.6 Application of a support (compression) bandage

foot with two further turns the bandage is taken round the ankle to overlap the heel section. Finally the bandage is spiralled up the leg, covering the paste bandage; the intention is to overlap on each spiral by half the width of the compression bandage itself. There are certain difficulties inherent in compression bandaging. The commonest fault is the production of a band of excessively high compression in the region of the calf. Subjectively the bandage should feel comfortable, and certainly not tight. Even if the pressure exerted by the bandage is optimal on application there will be a decline in the degree of support provided with time, principally as a result of movement by the patient. If the bandage slips it will be useless and may actually prove harmful. Finally there is the risk of sensitization occurring to the constituents of the bandage. There is no virtue in changing a support dressing frequently; a healing ulcer should be interfered with as little as possible. Reapplication is necessary when the bandage becomes loose, or soaked with exudate and malodorous. Application once or twice weekly is usually sufficient.

In view of these difficulties alternatives to compression bandaging are being tried. A tubular pressure bandaging system (Tubigrip) is becoming quite widely used. It produces relatively low pressures at the ankle but has a high degree of patient acceptability and requires minimal skill for application. To give the optimum control of oedema the Tubigrip should be applied first thing in the morning. If the ankles swell or become uncomfortable it can be removed by the patient and reapplied after a period of postural drainage. Tubigrip may be satisfactory but there is a risk that if it fits at the ankle it may compress at the knee. Two layers of shaped Tubigrip are advocated as providing a more satisfactory pressure gradient.

Elastic compression stockings are perhaps the most common treatment of all for chronic venous insufficiency. A variety of patterns, materials and styles are available. Appropriately fitted stockings will provide compression of 40 mmHg at the ankle. It is important that the compression be graduated, in other words the compression gradually decreases up the leg; support of this type will effectively reduce the ambulatory venous pressure. Compression stockings can be removed for bathing and at night. It is quite safe to sleep in the stockings but of course their haemodynamic properties are not required with the patient in the horizontal position. For the purpose of healing a simple venous ulcer a knee length stocking is normally sufficient, although some patients prefer full length stockings or tights. The 'Venosan' 2002/2003 and the 'Sigvaris' 504 are widely used and satisfactory. Materials for the yarn vary between manufacturers. The Venosan range are fabricated from a blend of nylon, cotton and Lycra. Lycra is a synthetic polyurethane elastomer which seldom causes sensitivity problems and is resistant to oils and perspiration. The stockings should not be applied directly to eczematous or ulcerated skin but they can be used quite satisfactorily over thinner dressings. Used correctly one can anticipate a life of 6–9 months for each pair of stockings. In cases of gross ankle–calf disproportion individual fittings of stockings can be arranged by hospital appliance departments who will also provide full instructions for correct usage.

If employed correctly there seems little doubt that either compression bandaging or elastic support stockings can provide sufficient graduated compression to enable venous ulcers to heal. There are so many subtly different regimes of treatment that direct comparisons are difficult to make. Selecting examples from the recent literature however we find a randomized trial showing that venous ulcers healed equally well with elastic stockings or a paste/elastic bandage regime[23]. In this study the stockings produced a slower result, although the graduated compression (24–16 mmHg) was lower than that usually considered optimal. A second randomized trial[24] compared a paste/elastic compression bandage with a hydrocolloid dressing applied under an elastic bandage that was removed every night. During the twelve weeks of the study there was no significant difference between the two groups at any time. My own view is that because of their effectiveness, simplicity and cosmetic acceptability elastic compression stockings are the most practical way of providing graduated support. They should be given long-term to all patients with healed venous ulcers. They can also be employed in many patients with active ulceration provided that the patients concerned can be taught to clean and dress their own ulcer on a daily basis. Some immobile individuals may find it difficult to remove the stockings and inevitably there will be some patients unwilling or unable to offer any active participation in their treatment. For these the compression bandage remains appropriate.

Systemic treatment for venous ulceration

In addition to the local measures described several drugs have been considered to have a place in the management of venous ulceration. Antibiotics, although frequently employed, have only a limited role. It is quite unnecessary, and indeed impractical, to think of 'sterilizing' an ulcer. A spreading streptococcal or staphylococcal infection can be very destructive and should be vigorously treated. Other than in these situations there is no evidence that systemic antibiotics aid ulcer healing.

Ulcers which are particularly offensive may be infected with anaerobic organisms of the *bacteroides* group. The use of metronidazole has been plausibly recommended under these circumstances. I think that it is premature to regard metronidazole as having an established place in the treatment of venous ulceration. In particular there is no evidence that ulcers so treated heal any more quickly. If an ulcer is excessively maloderous then the first step is to establish that this is not simply the result of inadequate dressing technique, or the presence of large amounts of necrotic tissue. If these possibilities are eliminated, and if bacteroides can be grown from the ulcer, a 10–14 day course of metronidazole would be reasonable.

Ascorbic acid and zinc salts have long been supposed to have a specific healing effect in chronic ulceration. A great deal of work has been performed on the zinc status of leg ulcer patients but without any very conclusive result being reached. High doses of ascorbic acid have been used for the ulceration associated with thalassaemia. Even relatively innocuous drugs cannot be employed without some risk. Some zinc preparations are nauseating. Patients with a high capacity to convert ascorbic acid to oxalate may develop renal calculi if treated with high doses of vitamin C. I doubt if either drug is beneficial in patients without actual deficiency states.

Conventional vaso-dilators have no therapeutic role in the management of venous ulcers. Recently, however, two drugs have aroused widespread interest. The bioflavonoids or hydroxyethylrutosides are a group of closely related chemical substances originally isolated from plants. These substances are marketed in the UK as Paroven. This drug reduces abnormal leakage from capillaries probably by an effect on the integrity of endothelial cell junctions. From current concepts concerning the aetiology of venous ulceration any agent that reduces fibrinogen leakage from dermal capillaries might be of therapeutic worth. Paroven has been shown to be effective in controlling the symptoms of venous disease such as aching, 'restless' legs, and night cramps. It also seems able to improve oxygenation of the skin in these patients. The results of a controlled trial assessing the ability of the hydroxyethylrutosides to aid ulcer healing is awaited with interest.

If the presence of a peri-capillary fibrin cuff is at least partly explained by impaired blood and tissue fibrinolysis then the use of an agent to stimulate fibrinolytic activity should be helpful. Such an agent would logically be given as early as possible in the development of venous disease. In a double-blind crossover trial of 23 patients the fibrinolytic stimulator stanozolol (Stromba) was compared with a placebo[25]. Both groups were provided with elastic support stockings. The authors estimated the areas of lipodermatosclerosis (a term they applied to eczematous, pigmented and indurated skin) and found that both treatment regimes reduced this. The combination of stanozol with elastic stockings was more effective although the degree of difference did not reach statistical significance. Stanozolol did improve the indices of fibrinolysis but most patients could not distinguish the subjective effects of the drug from those of placebo.

Because stanozolol may influence a critical step in the development of venous ulcers these results are of great interest. The study of venous disease of the legs is difficult and I wish that all agents marketed for its relief had received the close scientific scrutiny to which stanozolol has been subject. Nevertheless the results of further trials will be required before a final decision can be reached as to its place in the therapy of venous disease. The benefits observed in the trials reported so far must at least partially be attributed to the elastic stockings included in the regime. Indeed these could be the major factor responsible for the improvement. So far as I know nobody has yet claimed that stanozolol has any effect on existing ulceration although the drug may prove to be most valuable as an ulcer preventative. Against these prospects must be balanced some very definite problems. As an anabolic steroid stanozolol can produce acne, hirsutism and sodium retention. There is also at least the possibility of exacerbating pre-existing liver disease or prostatic carcinoma. Even the essential estimation of blood fibrinolytic activity by clot lysis time is not without its difficulties. Fibrinolytic activity shows considerable variability within the same individual and is easily influenced by such factors as physical activity. As things stand I think that the use of fibrinolytic stimulation is best confined to centres with experience in, and means of assessing the results of, the technique.

ISCHAEMIC LEG ULCERATION

The prevalence of symptomatic peripheral vascular disease in the UK has been estimated to be about 2–3% of men aged 45–60, and about 1% of women aged 50–65. Whatever the exact figures peripheral vascular disease is certainly the cause of a great deal of pain and despondency. In the elderly, in particular, the prognosis is dismal and the disease often unsuspected until a late stage.

Peripheral vascular disease is primarily atherosclerotic in origin and can present in one of three ways.

(1) Intermittent claudication;
(2) Acute arterial occlusion;
(3) Critical ischaemia (ulcers and pre-gangrenous changes).

The first two presentations are clearly the province of vascular surgeons but dermatologists may be involved with the third.

This is not the place for an exhaustive discussion of the aetiology of atherosclerosis. The currently accepted major risk factors are ageing, male sex, hypertension, smoking, diabetes and a strong family history. At a microscopic level the interaction between platelets and vascular endothelium seems of critical importance with the maintenance of endothelial integrity providing the protective barrier between the blood vessel wall and its environment. Platelet and endothelial homeostasis is maintained by the opposing actions of the vasoconstrictory and pro-aggregatory prostaglandin thromboxane A_2, and the vasodilatory, anti-aggregatory prostaglandin, prostacyclin. Once endothelial damage occurs lipids can enter the arterial wall although the exact mechanism is uncertain. As a result the uncomplicated atherosclerotic plaque forms consisting of the accumulation of extracellular lipid and cellular debris with smooth muscle cell proliferation. Later a complicated plaque may form with fibrosis, haemorrhage and calcification. The final event is mural thrombosis. The outcome for tissue supplied by an atherosclerotic artery depends on a number of patho-physiological factors. Perhaps the most important is the development of a collateral circulation both at the time of the acute episode and in the months following the acute stage. The presence or absence of vascular spasm and the rheological properties of blood may also be of relevance.

The management of ischaemic ulcers

The management of ischaemic ulcers is always difficult and it is unwise to give patients an over-optimistic prognosis. Many ultimately come to ablative surgery. As a preliminary cigarette smoking (though not alcohol) should be forbidden. Secondly any existing drugs taken by the patient should be scrutinized. Beta-adrenergic blockers should be used only with very great caution in patients with established peripheral vascular disease. More rarely ergot alkaloids can be the cause of problems. Investigations should be instituted to detect diabetes, hyperlipidaemia and polycythaemia. Since the only definite treatment for ischaemic ulceration is reconstruction of the leg arteries all such patients should receive the opinion of a vascular surgeon, and many will proceed to arteriography. Sadly many patients have distal disease which will not be amenable to surgical correction.

Regular cleansing of the ulcer should be performed. Although the benefits of topical treatment are very limited topical antiseptics, hydrogen peroxide cream, polymer powders or hydrocolloids have all been employed. I would normally select the material that the individual patient finds most comfortable. Whatever the material selected it should be held in place by the lightest possible dressing. Extensive skin necrosis can be produced by external compression if the cutaneous blood supply is compromised already.

It is essential that adequate analgesia is provided although it is frequently difficult to achieve without resort to the opiates. The use of buprenorphine sublingually can be valuable to cover painful procedures such as a change of dressings. Pain may dominate the clinical picture and many patients finally require amputation to control this intractable and distressing symptom. This procedure should not be delayed too long if efforts to salvage the limb are clearly hopeless.

Let us imagine a patient with ischaemic ulcers whose peripheral vascular disease is not considered suitable for surgical correction, but whose pain is insufficient to warrant early amputation. What courses of action are open? Three types of treatment have been used in this situation; lumbar sympathectomy, drug therapy and hyperbaric oxygen. We shall now examine each in turn.

Lumbar sympathectomy

Destruction of the lumbar sympathetic nerves can be effected by open operation or by an appropriately-placed injection of phenol (the so-called chemical sympathectomy). Lumbar sympathectomy is widely used in patients for whom arterial reconstruction is not possible. The place of the procedure in the treatment of peripheral vascular disease has recently been reviewed[26]. Skeletal muscle is innervated by sympathetic nerves but their effects are believed to be limited to resting muscle blood flow. During exercise, and even more during attacks of intermittent claudication, locally-produced metabolic products should already have produced maximal arteriolar vasodilatation. It has been suggested that sympathectomy might dilate collateral vessels and thus produce an increased blood inflow to the muscles. In fact large arteries are little influenced by sympathetic innervation, and the enlargement of collaterals that does occur is thought to be the result of gradual change in intrinsic smooth muscle tone.

Resting skin blood-flow is determined more by the demands of temperature regulation than in response to local metabolic requirements. Skin blood flow is regulated primarily by sympathetic control of the amount of blood flowing through cutaneous arterio-venous anastomoses. Effects of local heating and cooling are largely mediated by change in capillary flow, this being independent of sympathetic control. On the whole one would expect sympathectomy to have a beneficial effect on skin blood flow and ischaemic ulceration, but not on intermittent claudication. The outcome of sympathectomy is difficult to measure except in the extreme cases of eventual amputation or total healing of ischaemic ulcers. Modest subjective improvements in the degree of pain are notoriously difficult to quantify. No good large clinical trials of lumbar sympathectomy appear to have been performed and its adoption remains a matter of personal preference and experience.

Drugs in peripheral vascular disease

Numerous pharmacological agents have been employed in an attempt to reverse or ameliorate lower limb ischaemia. This topic has been excellently reviewed by Boobis and Bell[27]. There is no evidence that anticoagulants or anti-platelet agents have a beneficial effect on the healing of ischaemic ulcers. Beta-adrenergic agonists, such as isoxuprine, have no effects on skin vasculature. Alpha-adrenergic blockers, like thymoxamine, increase skin blood flow at the expense of muscle flow. Good controlled evidence of clinical benefits in patients with critical ischaemia of the foot is lacking however. It is even possible that they may do some harm if dilatation of responsive arteries 'steals' blood away from the diseased area. Nicotinic acid is believed to have a direct effect on skin vessels but despite many years of use its place is still questionable.

Rheological abnormalities have been noted in the blood of patients with lower limb ischaemia, notably elevated plasma fibrinogen and whole blood viscosity with reduced erythrocyte deformability. Attempts to lower blood viscosity by means of controlled defibrinogenation with pit-viper venom (Ancrod) have been made[28]. This technique produced some benefit to patients with intermittent claudication but the authors predicted that antibody formation to the Ancrod would limit the usefulness of the treatment to 6–8 weeks. This might be long enough to aid the healing of an ischaemic ulcer but the regime seems to be too complicated for use outside the specialist centres. Oxpentifylline (Trental) also decreases blood viscosity. The drug improves erythrocyte deformability and does appear to increase exercise tolerance in patients with intermittent claudication. Cinnarizine, a calcium antagonist, also has this effect. Naftidrofuryl (Praxilene) is described as a metabolic enhancer. It is intended to alter the metabolism of ischaemic cells so that they function better at the same reduced oxygen tension. There is evidence that used intravenously it may aid control of rest pain. It is sad to report that despite the novel approaches represented by these drugs their value in the management of ischaemic leg ulcers can at best be described as equivocal. So far as I know evidence that they improve ulcer healing rate is lacking and my own experience gives me no cause for great optimism.

Prostaglandins are naturally occurring fatty acids synthesized by cyclo-oxygenase enzymes from arachidonic acid. Two prostaglandins with circulatory effects have been widely investigated; PGE_1 (Alprostadil) and PGI_2 (Prostacyclin or Epoprostenol). Alprostadil relaxes smooth muscle and to a lesser extent inhibits platelet aggregation. It was first used in the treatment of severe peripheral vascular disease in the early 1970s. Its biological half-life is short since 80% of the drug is metabolized on first pass through the lungs. Because of this the first route selected for the delivery of this drug was intra-femoral arterial infusion. Prostacyclin is manufactured in arterial walls; it is a vasodilator and is extremely effective in preventing platelet aggregation.

In these respects it opposes the action of thromboxane which is synthesized in the platelets. In a small open trial Szczeklik and colleagues[29] gave a 72-hour intra-arterial infusion of prostacyclin to 5 patients with critical ischaemia of the legs. All patients experienced cessation of their rest pain and, in three, ischaemic ulcers healed within 2 months. Belch and colleagues[30] performed a double-blind trial on non-diabetic patients under 60 with ischaemic rest pain in one leg. They gave a 96-hour infusion of prostacyclin by the intravenous route. When compared with the controls 24 hours after the infusion the 15 patients given prostacyclin had significantly reduced rest pain and required less analgesics. In some patients these beneficial effects were still noticeable after 1 month. Although very encouraging these results are not strictly applicable to patients with ischaemic ulceration since the authors stated that they selected individuals with only very limited (less than 1 cm^2) skin necrosis. At present the prostaglandins are the most promising non-surgical treatment for ischaemic ulcers. Aside from the difficulties of administration these drugs have several unwanted effects including pyrexia, facial flushing and hypotension. Further large scale trials are now required.

In view of the difficulties and uncertainties associated with the use of drugs and lumbar sympathectomy it is hardly surprising that attention has been drawn to the possible use of other non-surgical modalities of treatment for ischaemic ulcers. Heng[31] and her colleagues devised a technique for administering hyperbaric oxygen using disposable polythene bags. The bags were sealed at thigh level and oxygen was then supplied at a pressure of 25–30 mmHg and at a rate of 15 litres/min. Treatment was given on four consecutive days each week for 2–3 weeks, or until the ulcers healed. Beneficial effects were dramatic. In the test group 18 out of 27 ulcers (5/6 patients) were healed in 6–21 days. The treated ulcers healed by 7.8% ± 1.15% per day. None of the five control patients showed worthwhile healing in a 3–7 week observation period. The numbers involved in the trial were small and the period of observation relatively short. Confirmation of these findings in a larger study would be a most exciting development.

THE TREATMENT OF OTHER TYPES OF LEG ULCERATION

There is universal agreement that diabetic foot ulceration is easier to prevent than to treat. The triple approach of good diabetic control, scrupulous foot hygiene, and regular expert chiropody is most strongly recommended. Infection, neuropathy and ischaemia are all involved to a greater or lesser extent in the development of diabetic ulceration; trauma may be the final precipitating factor. The treatment of established ulcers often requires a multidisciplinary approach in which endocrinologists, surgeons and dermatologists all play a part.

Pressure on the foot should be alleviated by bed-rest and the best possible diabetic control established. It is essential to reduce any oedema by elevation of the limb, and if necessary a course of diuretics. Early debridement of devitalized tissue is advisable and ulcer cavities and sinuses should be packed with chlorhexidine-soaked gauze. In this situation antibiotics have an important place and treatment should be instituted immediately under microbiological guidance. Simple neuropathic ulcers on the plantar surface of the foot may heal if a walking plaster-cast is applied with a window cut out to allow access to the ulcer itself. If conservative treatment fails a more radical surgical approach will be required. An early surgical opinion is particularly necessary if X-ray of the affected foot shows evidence of joint involvement or bony sequestration. Some type of limited excision may be sufficient but many infected, neuropathic diabetic feet ultimately require amputation.

The rarer problem of ulcerated necrobiosis lipoidica has been managed in a number of ways none of which is entirely satisfactory. Most patients are treated with simple dressings, but fibrinolytic stimulation and long-term inositol nicotinate have their advocates. Excision and grafting may be successful but there is a tendency for relapse to occur in the margins of the graft.

The weight-bearing surfaces of the foot have a limited tolerance of pressure. This is easily exceeded in any neuropathic patient whose feet are insensitive to pain. Any patient with a peripheral neuropathy should be taught the regular self-examination of feet and footwear, so that damage to the skin is avoided or at least is detected at an early stage. Established neuropathic ulcers can be treated with a walking plaster as already described.

In most other types of leg ulcer treatment follows on 'automatically' once an accurate diagnosis has been made. Sickle-cell ulcers will usually heal with bed-rest and conventional dressings. Excision and grafting would be the usual treatment for an ulcerated cutaneous malignancy. Ulceration associated with simple sepsis, or the more uncommon chronic infections (such as tertiary syphilis or a subcutaneous mycosis) should respond to appropriate systemic antimicrobial treatment. Pyoderma gangrenosum can result in rapid tissue destruction which in the early stages is easy to confuse with infection. It has been described in association with a variety of medical conditions and immunological abnormalities. Fortunately pyoderma gangrenosum normally responds to systemic corticosteroids; clofazimine and cyclosporin-A have been used successfully in resistant cases.

REFERENCES

1. Callam, M.J., Ruckley, C.V., Harper, D.R., and Dale, J.J. (1985). Chronic ulceration of the leg: extent of the problem and provision of care. *Br. Med. J.*, **290**, 1855–6
2. Cornwall, J. (1985). Leg ulcer specialist. *J. Distr. Nurs.*, August, 9–10
3. Perera, P. (1970). An investigation of varicose ulcers. *Trans. St. John's Hosp. Dermatol. Soc.*, **56**, 175–7
4. Yao, S.T., Hobbs, J.T. and Irvine, W.T. (1969). Ankle systolic pressure measurements in arterial disease affecting the lower extremities. *Br. J. Surg.*, **56**, 675–9
5. Black, M.M. and Walker, V.M. (1983). Basal cell carcinomatous change on the lower leg: a possible association with chronic venous stasis. *Histopathology*, **7**, 219–27
6. Peachey, R.D.G. (1978). Leg ulceration and haemolytic anaemia: an hypothesis. *Br. J. Dermatol.*, **98**, 245–9
7. Krull, E.A. (1985). Chronic cutaneous ulcerations and impaired healing in human skin. *J. Am. Acad. Dermatol.*, **12** (Suppl.), 394–401
8. Eaglstein, W.H. (1985). The effect of occlusive dressings on collagen synthesis and re-epithelialization in superficial wounds. In Ryan, T.J. (ed.) *An environment for healing: the role of occlusion*, pp. 31–4. (London: Royal Society of Medicine)
9. Silver, I.A. (1985). Oxygen and tissue repair. In Ryan, T.J. (ed.) *An environment for healing: the role of occlusion*, pp. 15–19. (London: Royal Society of Medicine)
10. Varghese, M.C., Balin, A.K., Carter, M. and Caldwell, D. (1986). Local environment of chronic wounds under synthetic dressings. *Arch. Dermatol.*, **122**, 52–7
11. Lookingbill, D.P., Miller, S.H. and Knowles, R.C. (1978). Bacteriology of chronic leg ulcers. *Arch. Dermatol.*, **114**, 1765–8
12. Eriksson, G. (1985). Bacterial growth in venous leg ulcers – its clinical significance in the healing process. In Ryan, T.J. (ed.) *An environment for healing: the role of occlusion*, pp. 45–9. (London: Royal Society of Medicine)

13. Dressings for leg ulcers (1986). *Drug Ther. Bull.*, **24**, 9–12
14. Brennan, S. S. and Leaper, D. J. (1985). The effect of antiseptics on the healing wound: a study using the rabbit ear chamber. *Br. J. Surg.*, **72**, 780–1
15. Ormiston, M. C., Seymour, M. T. J., Venn, G. E., Cohen, R. I. and Fox, J. A. (1985). Controlled trial of Iodosorb in chronic venous leg ulcers. *Br. Med. J.*, **291**, 308–10
16. Moss, C., Taylor, A. and Shuster, S. (1984). Comparative study of cadexomer iodine and dextranomer in chronic leg ulcers. *Scott. Med. J.*, **29**, 54 (Abstr.)
17. Katz, S., McGinley, K. and Leyden, J. J. (1986). Semipermeable occlusive dressings (effects on growth of pathogenic bacteria and re-epithelialisation of superficial wounds). *Arch. Dermatol.*, **122**, 58–62
18. Browse, N. L., Clemenson, G. and Thomas, M. L. (1980). Is the postphlebitic leg always postphlebitic? Relation between phlebographic appearance of deep vein thrombosis and late sequelae. *Br. Med. J.*, **281**, 1167–70
19. Burnand, K. G. and Browse, N. L. (1982). The postphlebitic leg and venous ulceration. In Russell, R. C. G. (ed.) *Recent Advances in Surgery (11)*. (Edinburgh: Churchill Livingstone)
20. Gowland Hopkins, N. F., Spinks, T. J., Rhodes, C. G., Ranicar, A. S. O. and Jamieson, C. W. (1983). Positron emission tomography in venous ulceration and liposclerosis: a study of regional tissue function. *Br. Med. J.*, **286**, 333–6
21. Goodfield, M. J. (1985). Platelets in gravitational disease; are they an aetiological factor? *Br. J. Dermatol.*, **113**, (Suppl. 29), 13 (Abstr.)
22. Dale, J., Callam, M. and Vaughan Ruckley, C. (1985). How efficient is a compression bandage? *Nurs. Times*, **Nov 16**, 49–51
23. Hendricks, W. M. and Swallow, R. T. (1985). Management of stasis leg ulcers with Unna's boots versus elastic support stockings. *J. Am. Acad. Dermatol.*, **12**, 90–8
24. Eriksson, G. (1986). Comparison of two occlusive bandages in the treatment of venous leg ulcers. *Br. J. Dermatol.*, **114**, 227–30
25. Burnand, K. G., Clemenson, G., Morland, M., Jarrett, P. E. M. and Browse, N. L. (1980). Venous lipodermatosclerosis: treatment by fibrinolytic enhancement and elastic compression. *Br. Med. J.*, **280**, 7–11
26. Lindenauer, S. M. and Cronenwett, J. L. (1982). What is the place of lumbar sympathectomy? *Br. J. Surg. Suppl.*, **69**, 517–23
27. Boobis, L. H. and Bell, P. R. F. (1982). Can drugs help patients with lower limb ischaemia? *Br. J. Surg. Suppl.*, **69**, 517–23
28. Dormandy, J. A., Goyle, K. B. and Reid, H. L. (1977). The treatment of severe intermittent claudication by controlled defibrination. *Lancet*, **i**, 625–6
29. Szczeklik, A., Nizankowski, R., Skawinski, S., Szczeklik, J., Gluszko, P. and Gryglewski, R. J. (1979). Successful therapy of advanced arteriosclerosis obliterans with prostacyclin. *Lancet*, **i**, 1111–4
30. Belch, J. J. F., McArdle, B., Pollock, J. G., Forbes, C. D., McKay, A., Leibermann, P., Lowe, G. D. D. and Prentice, C. R. M. (1983). Epoprostenol (Prostacyclin) and severe arterial disease. *Lancet*, **i**, 315–7
31. Heng, M. C. Y., Pilgrim, J. P. and Beck, F. W. J. (1984). A simplified hyperbaric oxygen technique for leg ulcers. *Arch. Dermatol.*, **120**, 640–5

3
CUTANEOUS BACTERIAL INFECTIONS

A. S. HIGHET

INTRODUCTION

This review concentrates on treatment. For biological and ecological aspects of human skin bacteria the reader is referred to Noble's *Microbiology of Human Skin*[1] and Maibach and Aly's *Skin Microbiology: Relevance to Clinical Infection*[2]. The relevant sections in Rook's *Textbook of Dermatology*[3] and Braude's *Medical Microbiology and Infectious Diseases*[4] are recommended for other clinical aspects such as aetiology, clinical features and diagnosis.

After some general considerations, topical antimicrobial agents are discussed in some detail. A similar treatment of systemic antibiotics is not provided as these are less specific to dermatology and are well covered in standard texts e.g. those by Kucers and Bennett[5], by Garrod, Lambert and O'Grady[6] and by Kagan[7]. I have not attempted to cover all possible therapies but I believe those included constitute a very full armamentarium. Acne, leprosy, the bacterial venereal diseases, infections which are primarily systemic, infections of burns, and some which are rarely encountered in the UK are excluded from the section on management of individual conditions.

GENERAL CONSIDERATIONS

Colonization and infection

Many bacterial species, including some which may be pathogenic, notably *Staphylococcus aureus*, can inhabit the normal human skin and may frequently colonize skin lesions. Therefore the isolation from skin of an organism with known pathogenic potential does not necessarily indicate a true infection requiring specific therapy. Conversely, it should be remembered that routine bacteriological investigation can occasionally give false negative results. The diagnosis of infection with the implied need for treatment, while sometimes difficult to establish with certainty in the context of secondary infection, therefore depends on an assessment of the clinical features in conjunction with – and frequently before the availability of – the laboratory findings. This is discussed in more detail in the section on infected eczema.

The role of antiseptics

It is sometimes stated, though usually not by those at the sharp end of clinical dermatological practice, that antiseptics will suffice for most superficial skin infections and that the use of antibiotics, especially topically, should be minimized. This is a sensible approach for secondarily colonized, or perhaps dubiously infected, skin lesions, but it is common clinical experience that in the management of established pyogenic infection with *Staph. aureus* and *Streptococcus pyogenes* antiseptics are inferior to antibiotics. The main value of antiseptics in clinical dermatology is in prophylaxis (including pre-operative cleansing), and in reduction of bacterial colonization of healthy or diseased skin. They may also reasonably be used as an adjunct to a systemic antibiotic and for continued or intermittent use after initial antibiotic therapy if recurrences seem likely.

Topical or systemic treatment?

Mild, superficial and localized infections may be treated topically, but systemic treatment is indicated for more severe, deep or widespread infections, any with lymphatic or systemic spread, and any involving *Strep. pyogenes*. If crusting is heavy, a topical antibacterial agent is advisable even if systemic treatment is also being used. Combined topical and systemic therapy may be preferred in severe or difficult cases.

Bacterial antibiotic resistance

The risk of the development and transfer of resistance may be especially marked with topical administration of antibiotics[8]. The duration of topical antibiotic therapy should therefore be limited to 1, or at the most 2, weeks; and antibiotics useful in major systemic bacterial infections should not be used topically, gentamicin being the prime example.

The high local concentrations achieved by topical administration of an antibiotic may overcome apparent bacterial resistance as routinely reported. Without testing against a wide range of antibiotic concentrations, however, this property should not be wholly relied upon and attention should be paid to laboratory reports of resistance patterns in conjunction with clinical assessment.

'Superinfection'

'Superinfection' with non-susceptible organisms is described as a complication of topical antibiotic therapy and that possibility is indeed an additional reason for limiting the duration of treatment. With short courses, however, superinfection is seldom a significant clinical problem except for candidiasis on mucosal and intertriginous surfaces, in which cases the inclusion of an anti-candidal agent will often be felt appropriate from the outset.

Contact allergy

Contact sensitization may occur with most topical antimicrobials, especially antibiotics but also antiseptics. Of the preparations discussed below, neomycin is the commonest sensitizer. Allergy to components of cream or ointment bases may also occur. As sensitization occurs most readily in lower legs affected by venous stasis, restraint in the use of topical applications is advised in that situation. Prolonged use predisposes to sensitization, another reason for limiting the duration of topical antibiotic treatment.

Steroid – antibiotic combinations

At the risk of tilting at derelict windmills, it is perhaps worth emphasizing the important place of these preparations in the management of infected eczema, especially of atopic type; one still occasionally comes across the attitude that such combinations represent sloppy practice. The case in favour has been well argued by Leyden and Kligman[9] and the question is further discussed below in the section on infected eczema.

TOPICAL ANTIBACTERIAL AGENTS

Antiseptics[2, 10]

Chlorhexidine is the first choice in most situations. It is active against *Staph. aureus*, *Strep. pyogenes*, and many Gram-negative organisms though not *Pseudomonas*, and maintains its activity relatively well in the presence of organic material and tissue fluids. Toxicity from percutaneous absorption has not been reported. It is colourless, only rarely sensitizes, and is largely non-irritant with the exceptions of the middle ear and the eye to which it should not be applied.

4% Chlorhexidine in a detergent solution (Hibiscrub) is probably the best such agent at reducing skin flora, and in addition to its widespread use as a pre-operative surgical scrub, it is commonly used in prevention of re-infection and cross-infection with *Staph. aureus* and *Strep. pyogenes*. The solution is worked into a lather on wet skin and hair and rinsed off; patients may need to be specifically advised that it is not a simple bath additive. The detergent may be irritant especially to atopic skin.

1% Chlorhexidine gluconate cream (Hibitane antiseptic cream) is inexpensive and clean. I commonly use it as routine prophylaxis after minor surgical procedures, though without proof of its value in this context.

0.5% Chlorhexidine in 70% ethanol is highly efficient at pre-operative disinfection of intact skin. 0.5% Chlorhexidine in isopropyl alcohol 70% with emollients can be applied (without rinsing off) to the operator's physically clean hands. There are surprisingly few combinations of chlorhexidine with topical steroids. Nystaform contains nystatin and chlorhexidine; hydrocortisone is added in Nystaform-HC.

Povidone–iodine is also a generally useful antiseptic with a broad antimicrobial spectrum, although the overall impression from the literature is that it is rather less effective than chlorhexidine. Significant systemic absorption can lead to hypothyroidism in neonates[11] and to hypernatraemia and acidosis if applied to large open surfaces. Its golden brown colour can be washed off but does place some limit on acceptability. Irritancy and allergy are uncommon.

In addition to the surgical scrub there are detergent presentations (e.g. Betadine skin cleanser) for washing skin and hair which may be tolerated by patients who find Hibiscrub irritant.

Quinolines have a wide antimicrobial spectrum, including activity against *Candida* and dermatophytes, and are most commonly used in combination with topical steroids. Measurable percutaneous absorption occurs and, though without proven hazard, may prompt caution in extent and duration of use especially in infants[12]. Sensitization is rare, though there are occasional irritant reactions. Their commonest presentations, as 3% clioquinol, stain skin and clothing yellow. However, potassium hydroxyquinoline sulphate 0.5% (with hydrocortisone 1% as Quinocort) and chlorquinaldol 3% (with hydrocortisone butyrate 0.1% as Locoid-C) are only minimally staining.

Silver is a useful agent against most bacteria including *Pseudomonas aeruginosa*. Silver nitrate in aqueous solution, commonly 0.5%, can be applied as a soak. Its absorption during prolonged administration to open or mucosal surfaces can lead to argyria and skin is stained black at application sites.

Silver sulphadiazine (Flamazine) is a much cleaner presentation, although bacterial resistance to the sulphadiazine component tends to emerge in long-term use. Contact allergy to the sulphonamide occurs occasionally.

Hexachlorophane is active against *Staph. aureus*, but it has been less widely used since the recognition that absorption can lead to neurotoxicity in infants.

Cetrimide has antiseptic and detergent properties. It is commonly used as an antiseptic shampoo, and alone or in combination with chlorhexidine as a skin disinfectant, although the resulting slipperiness of the skin can be a disadvantage for some procedures.

Ethanol 70–95% is a highly efficient skin disinfectant, alone or in combination with chlorhexidine or povidone–iodine.

Imidazoles, e.g. miconazole, have *in vitro* activity against Gram-positive but not Gram-negative organisms[13], though their main activity is against *Candida* and dermatophytes. Their value as antibacterials has yet to be confirmed in clinical use. Irritancy is an occasional problem but these drugs are clean and generally well tolerated.

Topical antibiotics

The earlier mentioned need, to minimize topical use of antibiotics important in treatment of serious systemic disease, should rule out *gentamicin* for all but the most exceptional and carefully considered topical use. Opinions have differed as to whether the same rigorous discipline should apply to fusidic acid; but the threat of multiple resistant strains of *Staph. aureus* argues in favour of restraint. Similar considerations do not apply to neomycin, bacitracin/gramicidin, polymyxin, tetracyclines or mupirocin, none of which has an important role as a systemic antibacterial.

Fusidic acid, if it is to be considered, is highly effective against *Staph. aureus* but less so against *Strep. pyogenes*. Its colourlessness, low propensity to sensitize, and low incidence of resistance are advantages. Its unique availability in gel form is tempting for scalp infections.

Neomycin is also very active against *Staph. aureus* and most Gram-negative organisms (though not *Pseudomonas* or *Bacteroides*), but has only weak activity against *Strep. pyogenes* and other streptococci. Allergic contact dermatitis can be severe but its incidence is acceptably low if its use is confined to short courses and avoided on skin affected by venous stasis[14]. This allergy extends to other members of the aminoglycoside group in a significant proportion of cases.

Neomycin may be absorbed through mucosal surfaces or inflamed skin so that application of large amounts may be ototoxic. However the maximum recommended dose[5] of 3 g corresponds to 600 g of a preparation containing 0.5% neomycin, a quantity unlikely to be exceeded in one course of treatment. For children 15 mg/kg per day should not be exceeded. Renal failure, however, may lead to accumulation of toxic levels from lower quantities applied. Resistance of *Staph. aureus* to neomycin is uncommon and is encountered mainly following inappropriate long term use; it extends to some other aminoglycosides but not gentamicin.

Neomycin is colourless and, perhaps partly because of its availability in combination with the stronger topical steroids, is perhaps the most widely used topical antibiotic. There is no longer, however, a simple neomycin–hydrocortisone preparation in the UK; Hydroderm contains also bacitracin but is available only in ointment form.

Bacitracin has good activity against *Staph. aureus* and *Strep. pyogenes*, less against other streptococci, and none against Gram-negative bacilli. Local reactions are rare and bacterial resistance is uncommon. Its availability is limited to combinations, e.g. with neomycin or polymyxin.

Polymyxin B has poor activity against Gram-positive organisms but covers nearly all Gram-negatives including *Pseudomonas* (but not *Proteus*). Acquired resistance is uncommon and topical use is safe. The drug is available in combination with bacitracin with and without neomycin.

Tetracyclines are highly effective against *Staph. aureus* and *Strep. pyogenes*. Reported resistance to either organism is, however, common, although in topical use the very high local concentrations may still be effective. Other streptococci, except Group B, commonly respond. Some Gram-negatives are susceptible but not *Proteus* or *Pseudomonas aeruginosa*. Tetracyclines are no longer vital drugs in major bacterial infections so that any increased resistance resulting from topical use, while undesirable, is not usually regarded as a serious problem. These drugs are well tolerated locally, allergy being uncommon, but their yellow staining properties limit their acceptability in many situations. Combinations of tetracyclines with steroids and nystatin are useful in short-term treatment of infected intertrigo.

Mupirocin (pseudomonic acid) is a new antibiotic highly active against *Staph. aureus* and *Strep. pyogenes* and some other bacteria (but not *Pseudomonas*). The claimed low propensity for the development of resistance, lack of cross-resistance with other antibiotic groups, absence of any systemic role, and good local tolerance are all admirable attributes for a topical antibiotic. Assessment of its value in clinical experience is awaited with interest but early impressions are favourable.

TREATMENT OF INDIVIDUAL INFECTIONS

The main primary bacterial pathogens of skin are *Staph. aureus* and *Strep. pyogenes*. The former commonly, and the latter less commonly, secondarily infect pre-existing skin lesions.

Staphylococcus aureus

Carriage

Staph. aureus is frequently carried on healthy skin.

With frequent sampling and special culture methods high rates of carriage (approaching 100%) are obtained, but with random sampling and conventional laboratory techniques the organism is found in the anterior nares in 35%, perineum in 20%, axillae in 5–10% and toe webs in 5–10%. Serial studies of nasal carriage show 20% of individuals to be colonized persistently, 60% intermittently, and 20% apparently not at all.

Systemic antibiotic treatment greatly reduces nasal and skin carriage of *Staph. aureus*, sometimes to zero levels, but recolonization occurs within a few weeks of stopping treatment. Topical agents are less successful perhaps because staphylococci on the turbinate mucosal surfaces are beyond the reach of digitally applied creams, although a reduction in numbers of bacteria short of eradication may be well worthwhile. Naseptin, containing neomycin and chlorhexidine, is frequently used in the short-term and long-term often without adverse effect, but neomycin resistance can emerge. My own practice is to use chlorhexidine cream alone for long term use, after a short course of Naseptin or an oral antibiotic if indicated.

Skin carriage is best treated by daily washing (including shampooing) with a chlorhexidine-detergent solution, with a povidone–iodine detergent preparation as second choice. Application of chlorhexidine cream to carriage sites may be a useful additional measure in difficult cases.

Suppression of carriage of *Staph. aureus* is indicated in patients suffering recurrent primary staphylococcal infections, classically furunculosis, and their contacts, as acquisition of a virulent strain is usually postulated. It would not usually be indicated in an isolated episode of staphylococcal infection without evidence of contagiousness in the household, and has an uncertain role in recurrently infected eczema in which the main abnormality lies in host susceptibility. Healthy carriers might require treatment by virtue of occupation, e.g. food handlers and operating theatre and neonatal nursery staff.

Systemic antibiotics in staphylococcal skin infection

Flucloxacillin, erythromycin or cephalexin would each be a good first choice.

The recommended adult dose of each of these drugs varies disconcertingly between 250–500 mg four times daily. The lower dose is often effective but I usually give the higher dose, at the cost of a higher incidence of gastro-intestinal symptoms, to larger patients, for more severe or recurrent infections, or where the lower dose appears to have failed.

Resistance to penicillin and, in many cases, tetracycline, is too

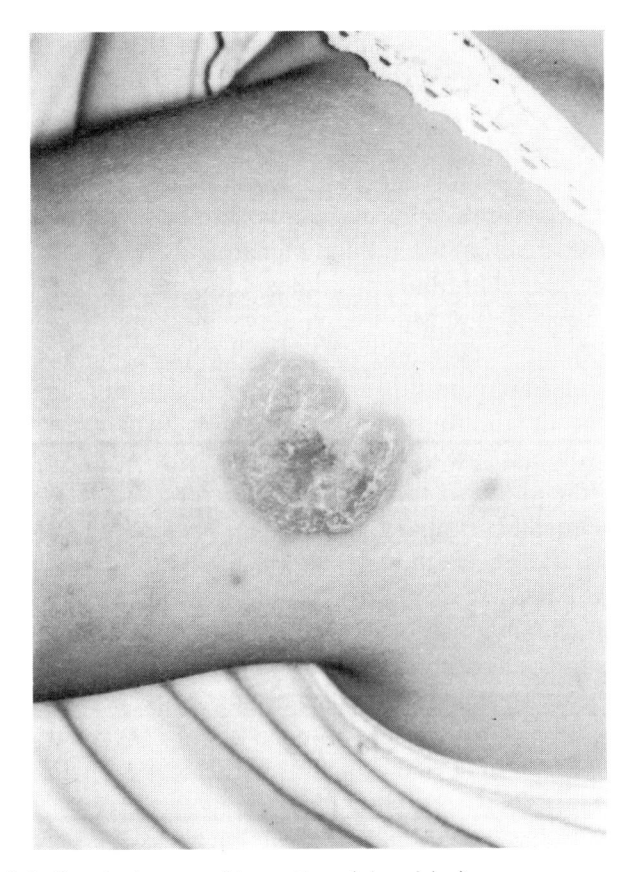

FIGURE 3.1 Staphylococcal impetigo (shoulder)

common for these drugs to be suitable 'blind' choices but if the organism is known to be sensitive these drugs would be satisfactory.

Impetigo

Impetigo is a superficial cutaneous infection with *Staph. aureus* (Figure 3.1), *Strep. pyogenes* (Figure 3.2) or both. The bullous form is exclusively staphylococcal. However opinions differ as to the relative importance of the two organisms in the non-bullous form, a dispute not

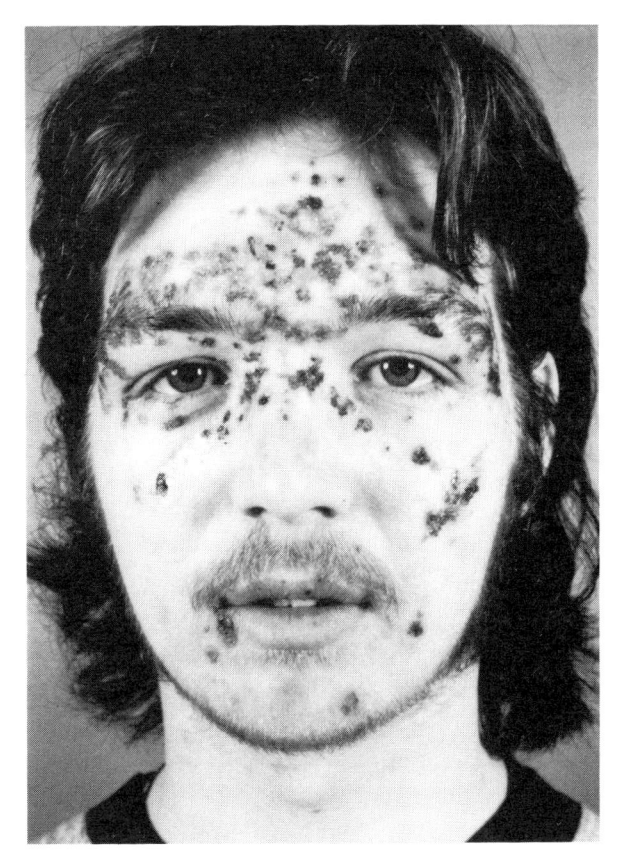

FIGURE 3.2 Streptococcal impetigo

necessarily readily solved by the bacteriologist in an individual case because secondary staphylococcal infection of a primarily streptococcal disease may suppress the streptococci. A pure staphylococcal impetigo is more likely in temperate climates and involvement of *Strep. pyogenes* in warmer climates. Heavy, 'dirty' crusts suggest the streptococcus. In practice it is not difficult to give treatment, topical or systemic, likely to cover both organisms and that is generally advised.

I treat most cases of impetigo with both systemic and topical antibiotics, although very mild localized infections, especially if *Strep.*

pyogenes has not been grown, will respond to an appropriate topical antibiotic. Antiseptics are acceptable if systemic therapy is used but would not alone constitute adequate treatment.

Topical neomycin or fusidic acid alone would be unsuitable if streptococcal involvement seems possible. A neomycin–bacitracin combination should cover both organisms; mupirocin may prove as useful; and the tetracyclines' yellow colour often seems insignificant on a background of disfiguring infected crusts. Ointments, at least in the early stages, are preferable to creams to soften heavy crusts which should be frequently washed and removed with soap and water.

Ecthyma (Figure 3.3)

The bacteriology and treatment are as for impetigo except that, because of the deep nature of the infection, a systemic antibiotic is always indicated.

Staphylococcal scalded skin syndrome

It has been said that once the epidermolytic toxin has taken effect, the value of antibiotics has not been proven, but few would withhold full dosages, given orally, or parenterally if necessary, of an anti-staphylococcal drug. General supportive measures and bland topical applications are also required.

Furunculosis

This staphylococcal follicular infection requires systemic treatment and a topical agent is also advisable. In recurrent cases carriage in the patient and household contacts should be sought and treated, and in

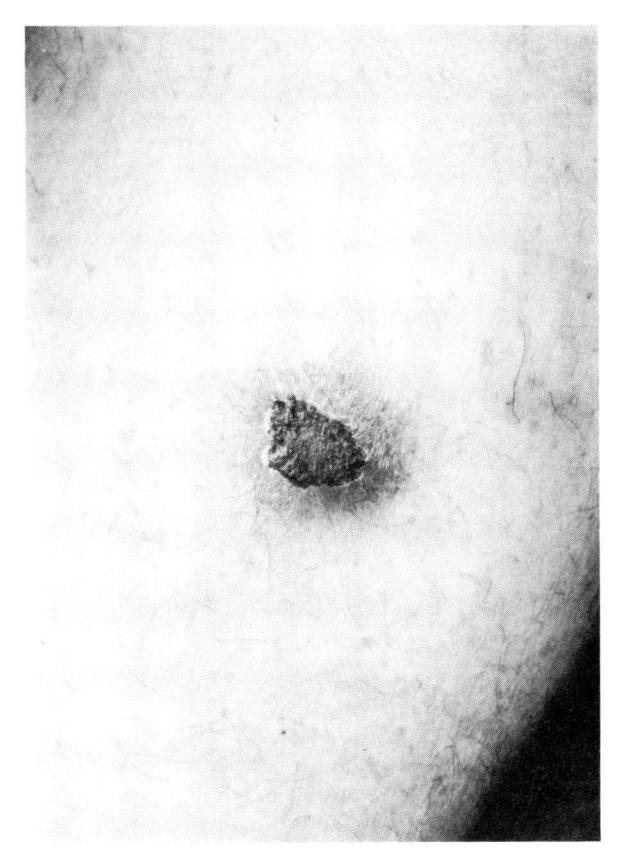

FIGURE 3.3 Ecthyma (lower leg)

difficult cases long-term (e.g. 2 months), flucloxacillin in half the usual dose may be justified.

Superficial folliculitis

This is not always an infective process; causative physical or chemical irritation should be avoided where relevant. An erythematous areola makes the pustule more likely to be staphylococcal. If the infection remains superficial washing and antiseptic creams may suffice, but any tendency to progress to deeper lesions would be an indication for antibiotic therapy.

Sycosis barbae

This scarring process begins with staphylococcal folliculitis which may become chronic or recurrent, requiring repeated or sometimes long-term antibiotics along with efforts to reduce staphylococcal carriage. A mild steroid in combination with a topical antimicrobial may help.

Folliculitis cheloidalis (acne keloid)

Staphylococcal infection should be vigorously sought and treated although in the late stages the condition is primarily one of scarring.

Acne necrotica

In this folliculitic scarring process usually affecting the temples and anterior scalp margin, staphylococcal infection should be pursued and eradicated. If this fails, long-term tetracyclines as for acne should be tried. The milder, generally non-scarring, acne necrotica miliaris is probably synonymous with *P. acnes* folliculitis of the scalp for which the treatment is long-term tetracycline.

Pseudofolliculitis

Inflammation results from penetration of sharp tips of shaven hair into the adjacent skin, either curling back if too long or penetrating the follicle wall directly if too short. Adjustment of shaving technique may be adequate but in those with curly hair, especially Negroes, the only certain cure may be to stop shaving. Any staphylococcal infection is secondary, although an antiseptic–weak steroid combination may help milder cases.

Streptococcus pyogenes (Group A streptococcus)

Strains carried in the throat in 10% of individuals are usually different from 'skin strains' and in any case tend to lose their virulence. *Strep. pyogenes* survives poorly on intact skin but readily infects even minor wounds. It is infrequently carried asymptomatically in the nose and on perianal skin. Attempts to eradicate such carriage with systemic antibiotics, antiseptic washing, etc are often unsuccessful but would be indicated if there is evidence of spread of infection to others.

Systemic antibiotics for Strep. pyogenes *infection*

Penicillin is the drug of choice and in severe cases may have to be given parenterally. Patients allergic to penicillin are usually treated with erythromycin. Tetracycline would usually be satisfactory if the organism was known to be sensitive. Oral flucloxacillin and cephalexin would be adequate in many cases, but none of these other drugs possesses the full activity of benzyl-penicillin.

Erysipelas and cellulitis

Erysipelas (Figure 3.4) affects mainly the dermis and upper subcutaneous tissue while cellulitis is a subcutaneous infection, so that depending on the level of infection the clinical pictures may merge.

Strep. pyogenes is the almost exclusive cause of erysipelas in the otherwise healthy host, and is the commonest cause of cellulitis although cellulitis may also be caused by other streptococci, *Staph. aureus*, and, especially in young children and on the face, *Haemophilus influenzae*, type *b*. Improvement in cellulitis is less rapid than in

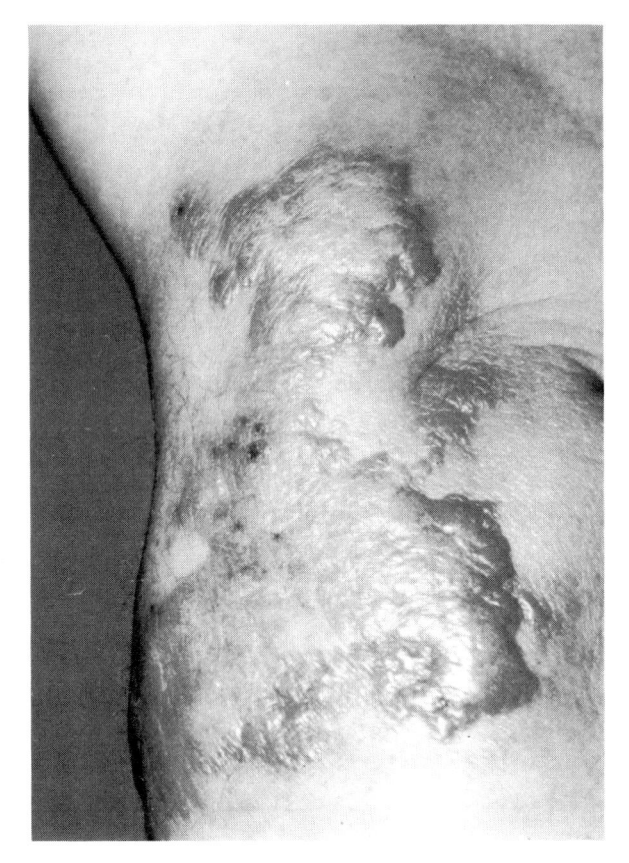

FIGURE 3.4 Erysipelas (arm)

erysipelas even on appropriate treatment, but a slow response to penicillin should arouse suspicion of a non-streptococcal cause.

Surface swabbing usually fails to yield the pathogen. In the immunosuppressed a wide variety of organisms may cause erysipelas and cellulitis; in these cases especially, blood cultures and even tissue biopsies should be performed in an attempt to isolate the organism.

Both erysipelas and cellulitis may leave residual lymphatic damage (Figure 3.5) which in turn predisposes to reinfection. Recurrent cases can be controlled by penicillin-V 250–500 mg b.d. taken for months or years and sometimes permanently. There is no definite point at which prophylaxis can safely be discontinued and the length of treat-

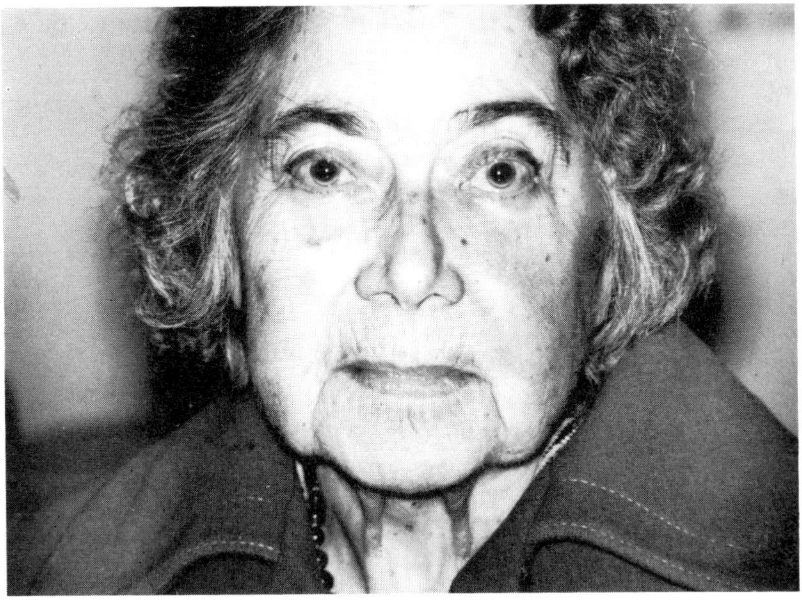

FIGURE 3.5 Chronic swelling of left cheek following cellulitis

ment will depend on the number and severity of previous episodes, whether recurrences develop rapidly on stopping the penicillin, and to some extent on the patient's attitude to long-term treatment.

Other antibiotics, to which streptococcal resistance may develop, would not be suitable for long-term prophylaxis. Patients allergic to penicillin should have a supply of an alternative drug, usually erythromycin, to take at the first sign of a recurrence.

Necrotizing subcutaneous infections

Necrotizing fasciitis is often due to *Strep. pyogenes* alone, but may also be caused by other organisms, singly or in combination, including other streptococci, *Staph. aureus*, Gram-negative bacteria and anaerobes. Early surgical debridement is nearly always required. Urgent Gram staining of the exudate will give some guidance as to the initial choice of parenteral, usually intravenous, antibiotics. One suggested combination is high dose flucloxacillin with clindamycin and an aminoglycoside.

Progressive post-operative bacterial synergistic gangrene requires similar management, but the disease is less fulminating than necrotizing fasciitis so that less extensive surgical debridement, and in mild cases antibiotics alone, may be adequate.

Erythrasma (Figure 3.6)

This superficial infection of intertriginous skin (including toe webs) is due to one or more aerobic coryneforms known as *Corynebacterium minutissimum*.

The imidazole creams (miconazole, clotrimazole, etc) are the usual first choice. Sulphur and salicylic acid cream and Whitfield's ointment are effective but often irritant in flexural skin. Fusidic acid is a useful alternative if its topical use is considered to be justified. Oral erythromycin is helpful in widespread cases. Relapses after treatment may occur, in which case antiseptic washes are indicated.

Trichomycosis axillaris

A variety of corynebacterial species cause the formation of sleeves of tightly packed bacterial concretions around axillary, and less commonly pubic, hair shafts, causing odour and staining of clothes.

Clipping of the affected hairs will help, along with topical antimicrobials such as imidazoles, sulphur–salicylic acid cream, Whitfield's ointment, 1% aqueous formalin and 1% clindamycin lotion.

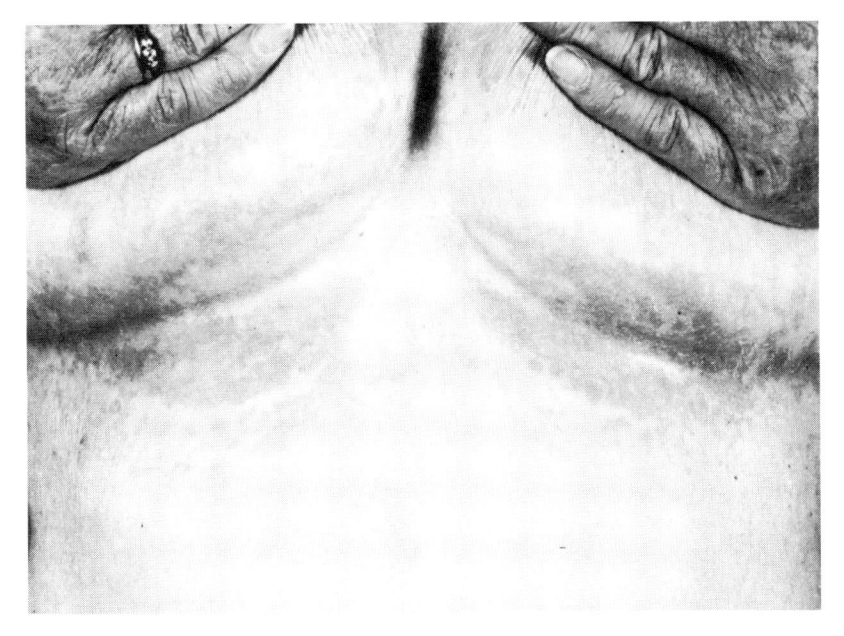

FIGURE 3.6 Erythrasma of inframammary skin

Pitted keratolysis (Figure 3.7)

This superficial probably corynebacterial infection causes well demarcated circinate erosions of the horny layer of plantar skin. Hyperhidrosis predisposes and should be treated but suitable topical antimicrobials include imidazoles and fusidic acid.

Erysipeloid

Erysipeloid is usually an acute but localized and self-limiting infection with *Erysipelothrix insidiosa*, often contacted through abrasions from animal and fish carcasses. Penicillin, tetracycline and erythromycin are each effective.

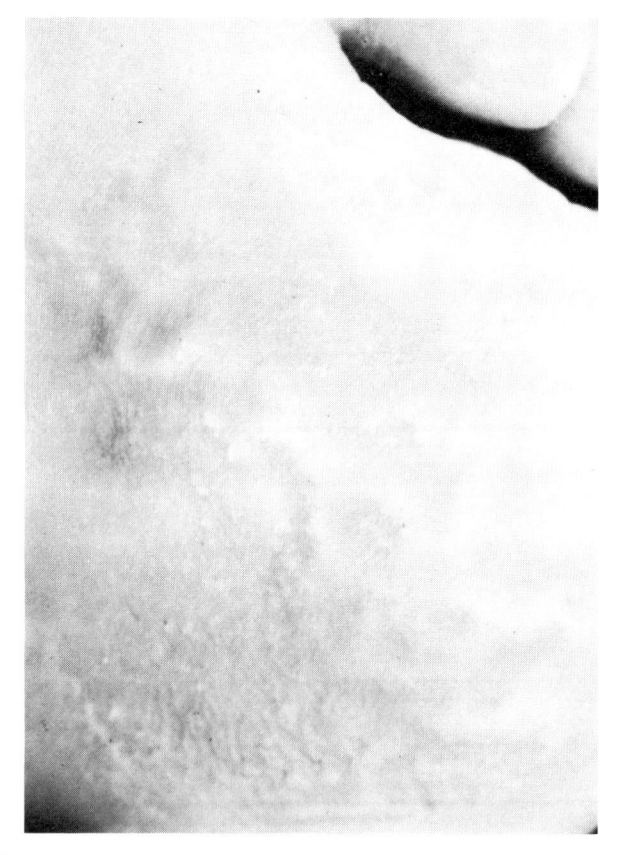

FIGURE 3.7 Pitted keratolysis (sole of foot)

Pseudomonas aeruginosa

Ps. aeruginosa frequently colonizes persistently moist habitats such as chronic leg ulcers without signs of pathogenicity. Potassium permanganate cleansing, exposure to air, and povidone–iodine soaks or dressings will reduce the numbers of, but often will not eradicate, the organism. If superficial pathogenicity is suspected a polymyxin-containing preparation (e.g. polymyxin–bacitracin (Polyfax) ointment, avoiding neomycin) or silver sulphadiazine may be tried.

Superficial and self-limiting folliculitis manifesting as itchy macules, papules, pustules and wheals may be contracted from bathing in water contaminated by *Pseudomonas aeruginosa*. Levels of chlorination satisfactory for cooler waters may be insufficient for the hot water used in often crowded whirlpools, a problem complicated by evaporation, and special attention must be paid to levels of chlorine and of pH for prevention.

From both such minor superficial types of involvement with *Ps. aeruginosa* mentioned above deeper necrotic infections may occur in the immunosuppressed requiring systemic therapy with a drug from the aminoglycoside, ureido-penicillin or newer cephalosporin groups.

Pasteurella multocida

This organism may cause deep infection following animal bites or scratches. Penicillin, ampicillin or tetracycline will be the usual first choice but patients with severe infection may require intravenous high dose penicillin or intravenous chloramphenicol.

Suppurative hidradenitis (Figure 3.8a, b)

This process affects apocrine gland follicles. The initial stages resemble acne but infection with pyogenic bacteria should always be sought. Once subcutaneous scarring and sinus formation occur, secondary bacterial infection often underlies exacerbations. *Staph. aureus*, anaerobic streptococci, *Bacteroides spp.* and *Streptococcus milleri* should be sought but bacterial involvement should not be ruled out on the basis of a single negative culture. Bacteriologically appropriate antibiotics should be given except that *Strep. milleri* responds poorly, in this clinical situation, to penicillins. Suitable choices for 'blind' therapy include erythromycin, or either minocycline or doxycycline, with possibly the addition of metronidazole.

Abnormalities of androgen metabolism in some patients[15] and the diagnostic and presumably pathogenetic significance of comedone formation raise the possibilities of antiandrogen therapy (in females)

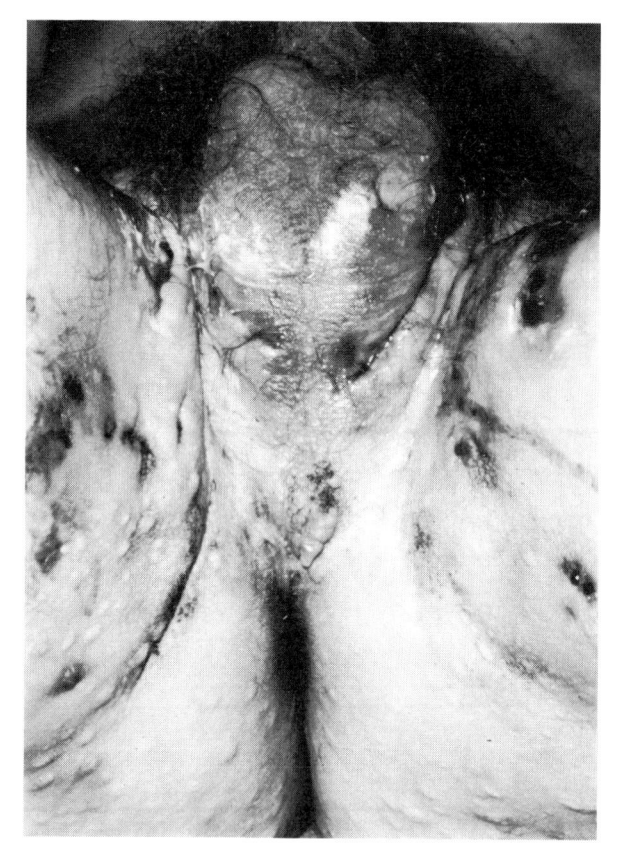

FIGURE 3.8 Suppurative hidradenitis **(a)** severe case in male perineum with actively discharging sinuses

and isotretinoin at least in the early stages of the disease but these measures have not to date been adequately assessed.

Long-term antibiotics, as in acne, may be tried but are often disappointing.

Advanced cases may require surgical excision which should be deep and wide.

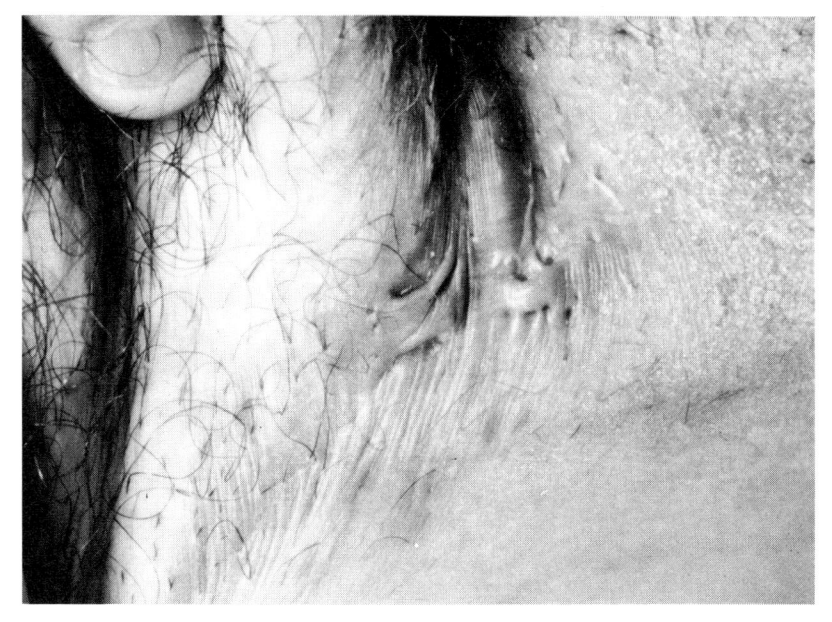

FIGURE 3.8 **(b)** mild localized lesions in female groin

Tuberculosis

Standard combination chemotherapy, for example as recommended by the British Thoracic and Tuberculosis Association in 1976[16], with rifampicin and isoniazid for 9 months with ethambutol for the first 2 months, will usually be required.

Internal or lymphatic involvement should be sought in cases of cutaneous tuberculosis, but where immunity is high, as in lupus vulgaris (Figure 3.9) and warty tuberculosis, the infection may be confined to the skin. In such cases some would treat with isoniazid alone, apparently without risk of resistance. Small lesions of lupus vulgaris which are not enlarging in an otherwise healthy patient may simply be observed, or may be treated locally by excision or cautery.

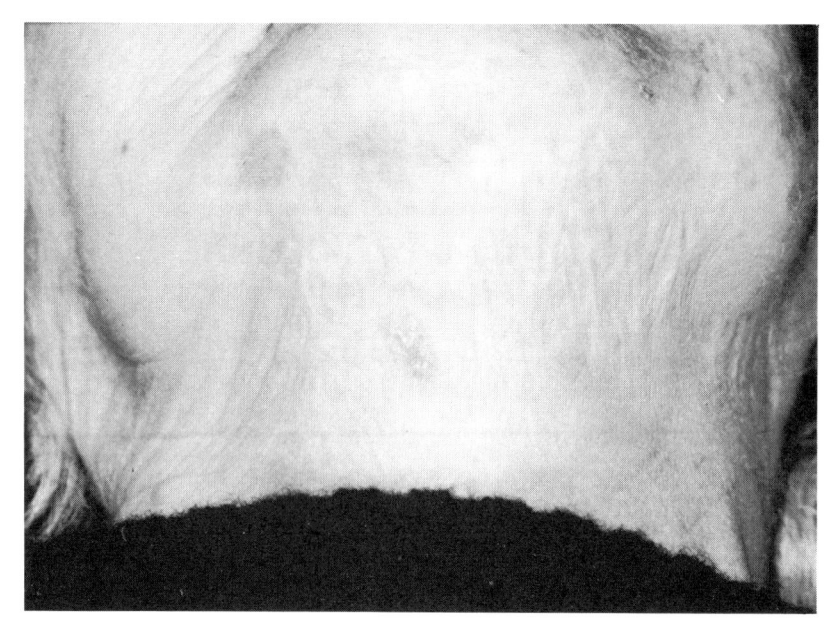

FIGURE 3.9 Lupus vulgaris under the chin with extensive scarring and a small central focus of activity

'Atypical' mycobacteria[17]

In all these infections sensitivity to antituberculous drugs and other antibiotics is unpredictable and should be determined in the individual case. Most are resistant to isoniazid.

The main form seen in the UK is due to *Mycobacterium marinum*. It enters damaged skin, often on the hand, from contaminated water including that in fish tanks and in inadequately disinfected swimming pools. Proximal lymphatic spread may give rise to a 'sporotrichoid' distribution of infected nodules (Figure 3.10). The lesions, though chronic, often eventually resolve and specific treatment may not be indicated. Rifampicin, ethambutol, cycloserine and ethionamide have been recommended. Some cases respond to minocycline, tetracycline or co-trimoxazole. Surgical excision provides the most immediately reliable treatment and curettage and diathermy are also effective, but the feasibility of these methods depends on the number, site and size of the lesions.

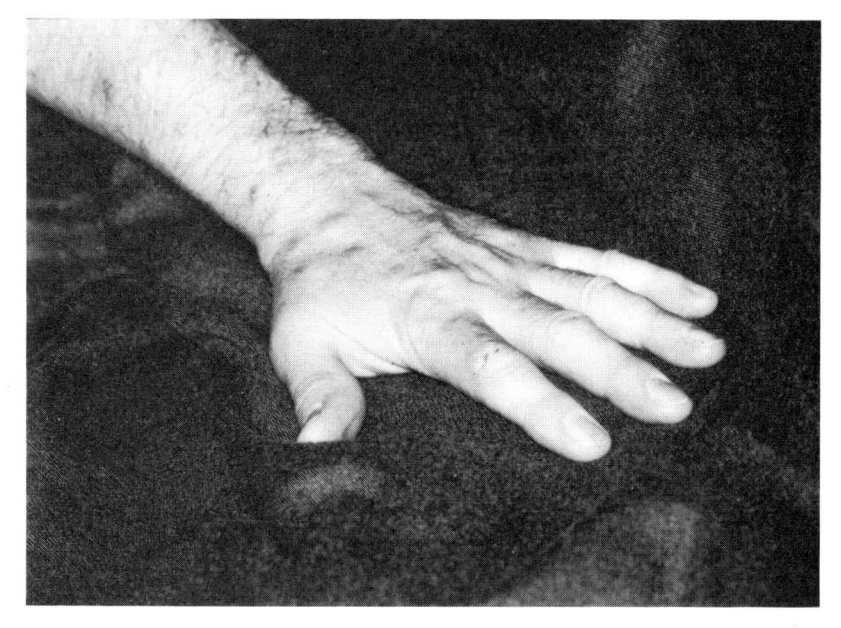

FIGURE 3.10 *Mycobacterium marinum* infection. The initial lesion is on the forefinger and the secondary nodules seen proximally represent the 'sporotrichoid' distribution

M. kansasii infections may respond to isoniazid, para-aminosalicylic acid and streptomycin irrespective of *in vitro* sensitivities.

Rifampicin is the main drug for *M. ulcerans* infections (Buruli ulcer) but is often disappointing. Treatment more often depends on surgical excision and grafting. Local heat and minocyline have each been successful in some cases.

The 'rapid-growing' mycobacteria, *M. fortuitum* and *M. chelonei*, may be resistant to all antituberculous and other antibiotics but the latter sometimes responds to erythromycin.

Chronic ulcers

These persistent moist lesions invite bacterial colonization. Whether actual infection is present is a clinical judgement, depending on signs of inflammation in surrounding tissues, deterioration in the ulcer itself, and systemic toxicity. *Strep. pyogenes* will usually be associated with cellulitis and require systemic treatment. *Staph. aureus* is much more commonly found, and while it may often cause enlargement of the ulcer or delay healing, many ulcers suffer no harm from its presence. Anaerobes will usually be associated with tissue damage and should be treated. Gram-negative organisms are very frequent but rarely seem pathogenic in the immunologically intact host.

A diagnosis of infection causing tissue damage will usually lead to treatment with a systemic antibiotic. I do not agree that topical antibiotics should never be used on leg ulcers, but the choice should be made for a definite indication; it is nearly always possible to avoid the commoner sensitizers like neomycin, and the duration of topical treatment should never exceed 2 weeks.

Uninfected ulcers may not require any antimicrobial therapy, the simplest and safest preparations being lukewarm physiological saline for cleansing and paraffin gauze or a dry non-adherent dressing (but not perforated plastic film which may lead to maceration of skin and increased bacterial growth). However, there is little objection to the use of broad-spectrum antiseptics routinely especially for ulcers which have been infected or heavily colonized. Iodine complexes are widely used and generally well-tolerated, including povidone–iodine 10% aqueous solution (e.g. Betadine) for cleansing, povidone–iodine ointment on a non-adherent fabric dressing (Inadine dressing; or extemporaneously with Betadine ointment on N-A dressings), and cadexomer iodine (Iodosorb) granules.

Bacterial infection in eczema

Any type of eczema can be secondarily infected, usually with *Staph. aureus* but occasionally with *Strep. pyogenes*, while the uncommon true infective eczema is directly attributable to bacterial infection. The management of these various forms of infected eczema is broadly similar, but here most attention is paid to the atopic type as infected atopic eczema is a common management problem and has been studied in most detail.

Significant rates of carriage of *Staph. aureus* on healthy skin have been referred to earlier. Carriage rates in general are higher on diseased skin. In atopic eczema 100% of exudative lesions, 90% of dry lesions, and normal-looking skin in nearly 80% of cases, yielded *Staph. aureus*, the density of organisms being highest in the exudative lesions and lowest in apparently normal skin[18].

Probably the main factor predisposing to *Staph. aureus* colonization in atopic eczema is mechanical disruption of the skin barrier function by scratching, though other factors may be relevant[19]. A pathogenic role for *Staph. aureus* is not doubted when there are clear clinical signs of impetiginization (Figure 3.11a) but there has been debate as to the significance of the isolation of the organism from lesions lacking such signs. Leyden and colleagues[18] produced evidence that organism densities below 10^6 per cm^2 did not appear to be significant, but that in an intermediate group with densities above 10^6 per cm^2 but below the very high levels of impetiginized skin, the staphylococcus appeared to be aggravating the eczema.

Antibiotics should be used in cases of atopic eczema with clinically evident infection, even if that is localized to a small area (especially around the ears and scalp) as widespread flares in the eczema can be associated with these apparently minor infections. Numerous small fissures in the lines of normal skin markings can indicate infection in the absence of purulent exudate and crusting (Figure 3.11b). In patients without signs of infection, the isolation of *Staph. aureus* in heavy growth on semi-quantitative culture, or failure to improve on other appropriate treatment, should lead to consideration of antibacterial therapy.

The choices between systemic or topical antibiotic or antiseptic have been discussed earlier. In the context of atopic eczema my own approach is broadly as follows. A definite or strongly suspected infection associated with deterioration in the eczema is treated for 1–2 weeks with an oral antibiotic and a topical preparation containing an antibiotic (commonly neomycin) and a steroid usually of higher strength than used by that patient in maintenance treatment. If infection has been frequent, a steroid–quinoline combination is tried after the initial course of antibiotics, and may be used long-term. If there are frequent recurrences sources of infection in household contacts should be sought and efforts made to reduce nasal and skin carriage (see earlier) in the patient. Detergent–antiseptic preparations may be tried (see earlier) but are often irritant to atopic skin. Applications of

(a)

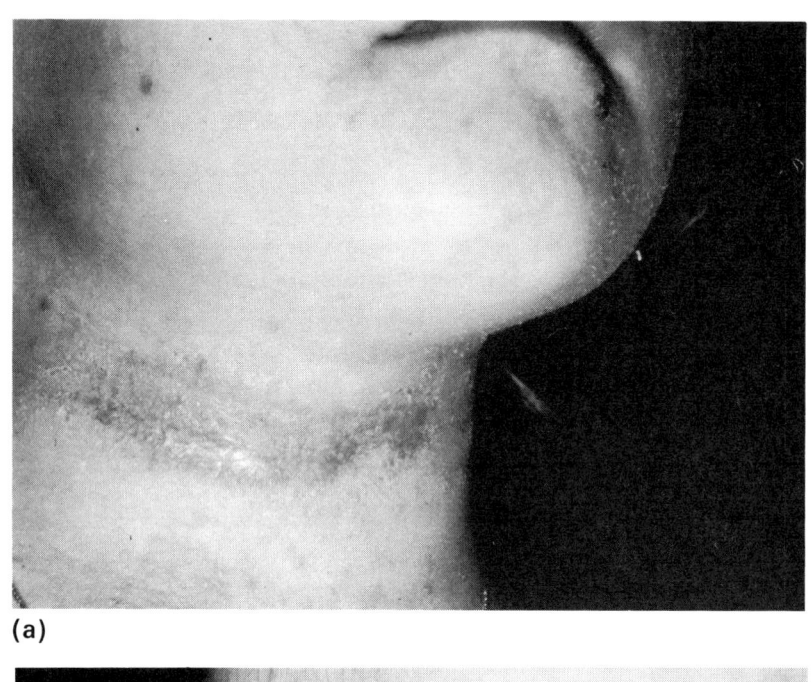

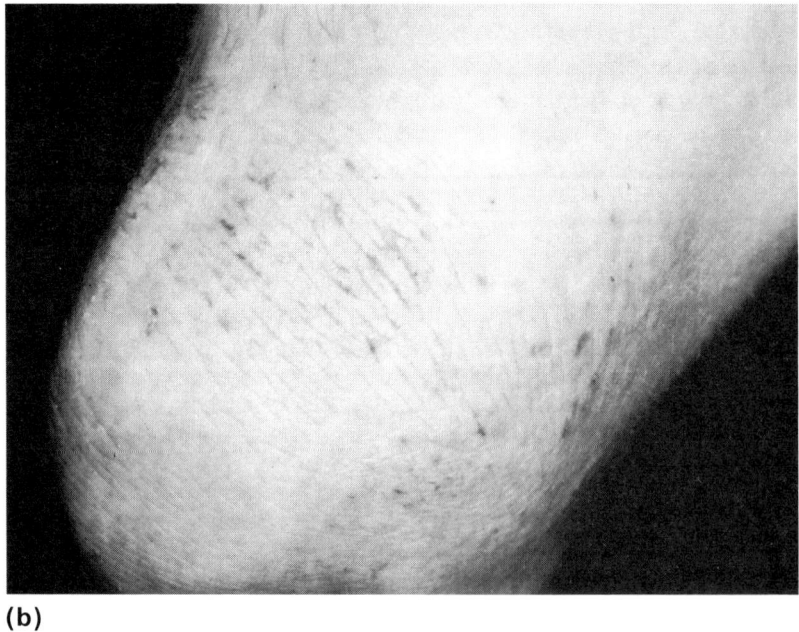

(b)

FIGURE 3.11 Infected atopic eczema (*Staph. aureus*) **(a)** impetiginized lesions **(b)** infection in small fissures on the knee

chlorhexidine cream after bathing with an emollient may help. It should be remembered that the infection is secondary and every effort should be made to deal with other exacerbating factors and to ensure adequate treatment with emollients and topical steroids. The better the eczema can be controlled overall, the less likely are further infections. Cases will, however, remain in which frequent pathogenic reinfection with *Staph. aureus* is a problem and, in those not allergic to penicillins, consideration should be given to long-term (for example 2 months) flucloxacillin in half the usual dose immediately following a standard course.

REFERENCES

1. Noble, W. C. (1981). *Microbiology of Human Skin*. (London: Lloyd-Luke)
2. Maibach, H. and Aly, R. (1981). *Skin Microbiology: Relevance to Clinical Infection*. (New York: Springer-Verlag)
3. Rook, A. J., Wilkinson, D. S., Ebling, F. J. G., Champion, R. H. and Burton, J. L. (eds.) (1986). *Textbook of Dermatology* 4th Edn. (Oxford: Blackwell)
4. Braude, A. I. (1981). *Medical Microbiology and Infectious Diseases*. (Philadelphia: Saunders)
5. Kucers, A. and Bennett, N. McK. (1979). *The Use of Antibiotics* 3rd Edn. (London: Heinemann)
6. Garrod, L. P., Lambert, H. P. and O'Grady, F. (1981). *Antibiotic and Chemotherapy* 5th Edn. (Edinburgh: Churchill Livingstone)
7. Kagan, B. M. (1980). *Antimicrobial Therapy* 3rd Edn. (Philadelphia: Saunders)
8. Noble, W. C. and Naidoo, J. (1978). Evolution of antibiotic resistance in *Staphylococcus aureus:* the role of the skin. *Br. J. Dermatol.*, **98,** 481–9
9. Leyden, J. J. and Kligman, A. M. (1977). The case for steroid–antibiotic combinations. *Br. J. Dermatol.*, **96,** 179–87
10. Sebben, J. E. (1983). Surgical Antiseptics. *J. Am. Acad. Dermatol.*, **9,** 759–65
11. Jackson, H. J. and Sutherland, R. M. (1981). Effect of povidone-iodine on neonatal thyroid function. *Lancet*, **2,** 992
12. Stohs, S. J., Ezzedeen, F. W., Anderson, A. K. *et al.* (1984). Percutaneous absorption of iodochlorhydroxyquin in humans. *J. Invest. Dermatol.*, **82,** 195–8
13. Sud, I. J. and Feingold, D. S. (1982). Action of antifungal imidazoles on *Staphylococcus aureus*. *Antimicrob. Agents Chemother.*, **22,** 470–4
14. MacDonald, R. H. and Beck, M. (1983). Neomycin: a review with particular reference to dermatological use. *Clin. Exp. Dermatol.*, **8,** 249–58
15. Mortimer, P. S., Dawber, R. P. R., Gales, M. A. *et al.* (1986). Mediation of hidradenitis suppurativa by androgens. *Br. Med. J.*, **292,** 245–8
16. British Thoracic and Tuberculosis Association. (1976). Short-course chemotherapy in pulmonary tuberculosis. *Lancet*, **2,** 1102–4
17. Beyt, B. E., Ortbals, D. W., Santa Cruz, D. J. *et al.* (1980). Cutaneous myco-

bacteriosis: analysis of 34 cases with a new classification of the disease. *Medicine (Baltimore)*, **60,** 95–109
18. Leyden, J. J., Marples, R. R. and Kligman, A. M. (1974). *Staphylococcus aureus* in the lesions of atopic dermatitis. *Br. J. Dermatol.*, **90,** 525–30
19. Dahl, M. V. (1983). *Staphylococcus aureus* and atopic dermatitis. *Arch. Dermatol.*, **119,** 840–6

4
URTICARIA

R. P. WARIN

Urticaria (hives or nettle rash) may be described as an eruption of transient circumscribed oedematous and usually itchy swellings in the dermis, which usually last for a few hours up to 48 hours and then clear, leaving clinically normal skin. Angioedema (giant urticaria) is the exact counterpart but involves the subcutaneous tissues. Table 4.1 gives the different patterns of urticaria and their approximate incidence in hospital practice.

ACUTE URTICARIA

Acute attacks of urticaria may be due to an allergic response to a drug, food or infective agent such as hepatitis, glandular fever and also parasites. However in the majority of cases the cause is not determined. Attacks often last 1–2 days but sometimes they persist and in a few cases, drag on for weeks and may merge into chronic urticaria, which is artificially defined as urticaria lasting more than 6–8 weeks. Whatever the cause the clinical appearance is similar with the whole range of small and large weals and angioedema swellings. The edges of weals may spread but clearing in the centre gives an appearance of rings and arcuate lesions (Figure 4.1). Individual weals last a few hours but particularly with angioedema swellings they may not completely fade for 2–3 days. Painful and at times swollen joints may accompany the attack.

TABLE 4.1 Patterns of urticaria

	Percentage incidence
Ordinary urticaria Acute / Chronic / Angioedema	72
Urticarial vasculitis	5
Physical urticaria	
Dermographism	10
Cholinergic (exercise, heat)	6
Cold	3
Aquagenic, direct heat, solar, etc	1
Deep pressure	2
Hereditary angioedema	1

Other types of urticaria include contact urticaria, stings and bites (papular urticaria) and urticaria pigmentosa.

A careful history may suggest a cause and, for example, in the case of food, this can be followed up by avoidance, challenge tests and in a few cases, such as for example, nut allergy, a prick test may help to confirm the diagnosis. A blood count showing an eosinophilia would indicate further investigations in connection with possible parasitic infestation. It is quite common to get recurrences associated with upper respiratory tract infections unrelated to any treatment. Acute attacks may be recurrent even without an obvious precipitating cause.

In the usual case the course is self-limited and therapy directed only to symptomatic relief. H1 antagonists will undoubtedly help and usually relieve most of the itching. In some severe attacks the stimulus to weal production is so severe that the effect of even large doses of antihistamines may appear slight. In acute attacks the antihistamine may be given by intramuscular injection but it must be remembered that the 1–2 hours delay in reaching 50% action is largely due to the

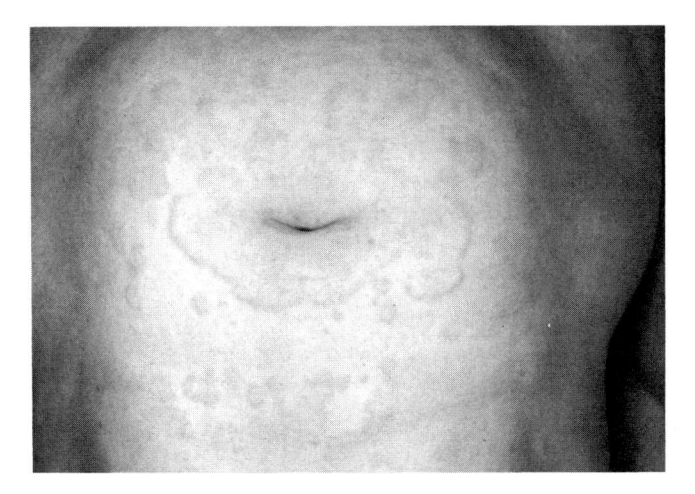

FIGURE 4.1 Annular and spreading weals in acute urticaria

time taken for the antagonist to become fixed on the cells and the absorption delay is comparatively slight.

If an associated angioedema is severe or there are serious anaphylactic complications, the immediate treatment is with epinephrine, 0.5–1.0 ml of the 1:1000 preparation intramuscularly and 0.5 ml repeated every 20–30 minutes if necessary. In very severe attacks corticosteroid therapy may also be indicated, perhaps starting with a dose of prednisolone of 40 mg in the first 24 hours, which can then be reduced over the next 1–2 weeks.

CHRONIC URTICARIA

The first problem in the management of chronic urticaria is one of diagnosis. A common difficulty is differentiating chronic urticaria from a physical urticaria. Apart from determining the physical cause from the history and by simple tests, weals and larger swellings last a much shorter time of $\frac{1}{2}$–1 hour (excluding deep pressure urticaria), whereas in chronic urticaria the weals usually last for 3–8 hours or longer. The causative physical factor is often not recognized by the patient, particularly unnoticed friction from clothing and furniture may start up a dermographic weal which is then thought by the patient to be spontaneous. One important aspect of distinguishing a physical urticaria from chronic urticaria is that in the former the whole range of drug and food allergy causes do not play any part, with the possible exception of an aspirin reaction in cholinergic urticaria.

Although eczematous dermatitis reactions will leave scaling, this feature may not be apparent when the patient is examined between recurrent attacks and urticaria could be wrongly diagnosed. The size and shape of weals varies considerably but the significance of these variations is not apparent. There is one type of chronic urticaria which always produces small weals of up to 2–4 mm diameter and this can be confused with cholinergic urticaria, although in this chronic urticaria the weals will last for much longer and not be associated with the precipitating factors of heat and exercise (Figure 4.2). Drugs, food and infective agents, including fungi and parasites, may be

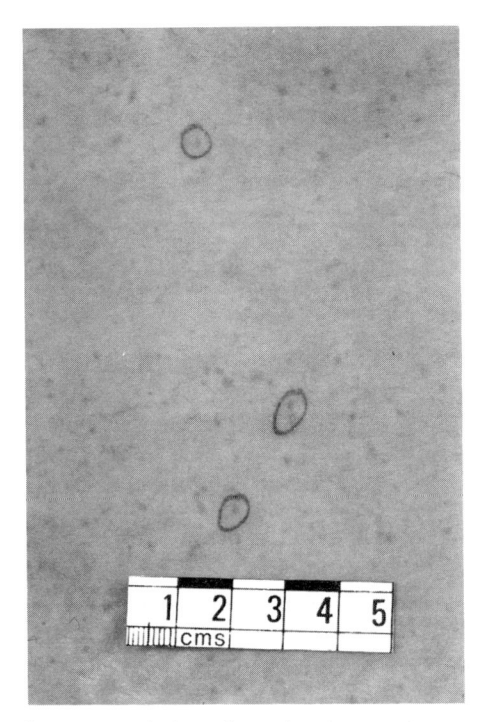

FIGURE 4.2 Small patterned chronic urticaria

pinpointed as the cause, but in at least 80% of patients with chronic urticaria the essential cause is not clear[1]. Amongst drug causes penicillin must be mentioned. Penicillin and related antibiotics are common causes of acute urticaria and at one time it was considered that small amounts of penicillin contaminating foods such as dairy products were the cause of some cases of chronic urticaria. Nowadays the amount of penicillin in milk is negligible and in spite of the study of Boonk and van Ketel[2] it seems likely that this cause is extremely rare. Dietary yeast and intestinal candidiasis can occasionally be a cause and it is worthwhile performing an intradermal test to candida albicans because if positive, a course of nystatin and a low-yeast diet may well help[3]. A blood count may show an eosinophilia which raises the possibility of parasitic infection. A raised ESR, complement abnormalities and auto-immune tests are relevant in relation to urticarial vasculitis. Other tests may be indicated by the general examination, for example if there is evidence of cholecystitis or thyroid disorders.

There often appear to be a number of inter-related factors and although not the main cause, various agents can increase the urticarial tendency and give rise to exacerbations. For example, some 30–40% of patients with chronic urticaria will have exacerbations after taking salicylates if given in large enough doses, and it is, therefore, important to advise patients to avoid aspirin-containing preparations[4] (Figure 4.3). Apart from salicylates, azo dyes, benzoic acid preservatives, yeasts and probably other substances may have a similar effect[5]. It is important to determine whether these exacerbating factors are operative in an individual case, as their removal through dietary control is often enough to cause the urticaria to settle down[6]. Various dietary investigations have been elaborated, ranging from simple avoidance of substances, to keeping a food diary and the use of an elimination diet when simple foods are given and various foods added at intervals of a few days. However, a more practical way of determining whether such factors are playing a part is to give test doses of the various substances likely to be involved, over a period of days (e.g. tartrazine 10 mg, sodium benzoate 500 mg, aspirin 100 mg). Because of the vagaries of chronic urticaria it is essential to give the substances in unmarked identical capsules, interspersed with inert control capsules, as a 'challenge test battery'. It is interesting that patients who have shown exacerbations to substances when their phase of urticaria is active,

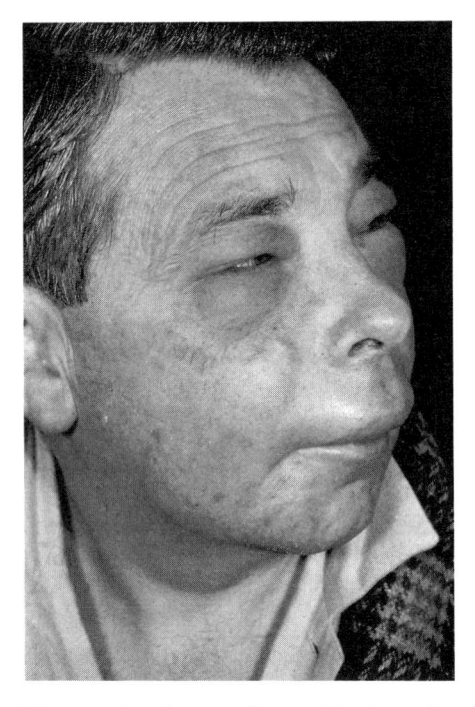

FIGURE 4.3 Aspirin reaction in a patient with chronic urticaria

may well be able to take them without trouble once the urticaria tendency has settled down[7].

Frequently there is a constitutional and nervous factor and patients pass through phases when the urticaria is present and these times may well coincide with difficult or stressful periods in their lives. Certain times in life are associated with periods of urticaria, for example, the menopause and premenstrually in women. It has often been thought that this latter association was a secondary effect of the increased tension which may occur at this time but changes in fluid balance and in blood vessels premenstrually are complex and might well have some action on an underlying urticarial tendency. A progesterone sensitivity has been suggested as a cause but would hardly apply to such a common phenomenon as urticaria. Similarly urticaria may develop during pregnancy and may reappear in subsequent pregnancies. 'Suggestion' plays an important part in the treatment of chronic urticaria and undoubtedly patience by the physician is often rewarding. Many cases of chronic urticaria last for a period of 6–12 months and then naturally settle down. Obviously the treatment at that point will erroneously be acclaimed as successful. In severe cases and in those where the physician and patient are becoming desperate, admission to hospital will often cause urticaria to clear.

Drug treatment of chronic urticaria

H1 antagonists

Since 1948 H1 antagonists have been the sheet anchor of drug treatment in chronic urticaria. Most patients are helped to some extent and itching often reduced. In some severe cases and during exacerbations, the effect of the H1 antagonists may appear slight, whereas in some patients often with a milder condition, the weals can be completely suppressed.

In the past the main problem has been the side-effects of the H1 antagonists, particularly drowsiness, and much of the art of treatment was to administer different antihistamines and arrange the drug routine with the idea of minimizing the side-effects. In the last few years terfenadine and more recently astemizole have been introduced and the incidence of drowsiness with these substances is no greater than that complained of when placebo drugs are given. These introductions have revolutionized antihistamine therapy and probably the only justification for using the older antihistamines is if a slight sedative effect is deliberately sought. For example, brompheniramine maleate 12 mg at night may help to reduce weals during the night and also promote sleep, and apart from the early morning, usually gives no daytime drowsiness. Hydroxyzine hydrochloride can also be used in a similar way. Weight gain has been described in the past particularly with cyproheptadine and this change may occur with terfenadine and astemizole, particularly the latter. A reducing diet may be sufficient to control this curious complication. Because of the absence of drowsiness with terfenadine, it has been possible to give large doses. However it has been found that doses greater than double or treble the usual dose of terfenadine (which is 120 mg daily), give no more effect, presumably because mediators other than those which can be inhibited by H1 antagonists play an important part in urticarial weal production.

The H1 antagonists all have other pharmacological actions, such as an antiserotonin effect in some, and there has been an attempt in the past to link these with their use in certain types of urticaria. There is, however, no clear-cut evidence that these other pharmacological actions are of benefit.

H2 antagonists

Cimetidine and ranitidine have little effect on weal size, but when added to H1 antagonists there is a slightly greater effect on the induced histamine weal and the weal of dermographism[8]. There is some debate as to the value of adding H2 antagonists to H1 antagonists in patients with chronic urticaria, but it would seem that this is rarely of much benefit in practical management[9,10].

Other drugs

Beta-adrenergic agents such as adrenalin are helpful in severe attacks and ephedrine has a place in management of difficult urticaria. Terbutaline is another beta-adrenergic drug which has been used alone or in combination with ketotifen. Results have varied but Saihan[11] had some success in patients with refractory urticaria. A common and distressing side-effect of terbutaline is tremor of the limbs. The cromoglycate-like drugs have also been tried but with no regular success and oxatomide and ketotifen both with multiple properties including cromoglycate-like effects, have not been generally effective; both can cause drowsiness.

Tricyclic anti-depressants are known to exert a potent H1 antagonist effect. Amitriptyline and doxepin have been used in patients with chronic urticaria with good results, particularly if there has been some underlying depression. Systemic corticosteroids will reduce the wealing in most patients but as treatment often needs to be continued for a long period, serious side-effects develop. They do have a place in special situations and in order to gain control in severe and resistant cases.

Although most cases of urticaria settle down after a few months, all dermatologists have to struggle with the small group of patients with chronic urticaria, which continues for years. As would be expected all sorts of drugs have been used and go in and out of fashion, but the desperate physician may well want to try these miscellaneous treatments, which range from auto-haemotherapy to calcium gluconate, heparin and menaphthone. As tranexamic acid was of great benefit in angioedema, this has also been used in chronic urticaria with a few successful claims.

ANGIOEDEMA

Although angioedema swellings occur commonly in association with both acute and chronic urticaria, there are a few patients who have recurrent angioedema with no or very insignificant urticarial weals[12]. In patients with recurrent angioedema it is, of course, important to exclude an intermittently-taken drug or food. There is also a group of patients with this condition associated with fever and high eosinophilia, which has been recently described[13].

The differential diagnosis of recurrent angioedema can be very difficult, as the patients are often seen in a quiescent phase and the diagnosis has to be made on historical data. Recurrent attacks of contact dermatitis, due to primula for example, can be difficult to exclude because the scaling remaining after the attack may have cleared or not be noticed. Contact urticaria from, for example, close association with cats, dogs or horses can also be difficult. The physical urticarias can be associated with deeper swellings and for example, rubbing the eyelids in a patient with dermographism will cause swelling as will pressure from the teeth on the lips. Similarly swelling of the eyelids can occur with severe attacks of cholinergic urticaria.

Once angioedema has developed it is probably not affected by H1 antagonists. If the attacks are occurring frequently it may be worthwhile taking an antihistamine regularly over long periods and this is now quite easy by virtue of the new non-sedative antihistamines. In acute very severe angioedema adrenalin by injection may well help.

URTICARIAL VASCULITIS

In the past 1–2% of patients with urticaria have been said to have a vasculitis on histology, including patients with systemic lupus erythematosus (Figure 4.4). It is now known that a greater percentage show changes of leucocytoclastic vasculitis and various recent series report an incidence of 5%. However if the histo-pathological criteria for diagnosis of vasculitis are less rigorous, then some 20% or even 40% with urticaria will show some changes suggesting vasculitis[14]. Indeed as pointed out by Russell Jones *et al.*[15] there is a continuum of changes from obvious leucocytoclastic vasculitis to patients showing slight or no evidence of these changes.

In severe grades of urticarial vasculitis weals tend to last longer, may even be present for 2–3 days and leave purpuric staining. Otherwise the eruption cannot be clinically distinguished. There is a small group of patients with vasculitis who also have a complement abnormality and some cases have joint and renal involvement[16]. Urticarial vasculitis responds well to systemic corticosteroids but large doses are often necessary and the treatment has to be continued for a long period. Even in the face of vasculitis H1 antagonists help to some extent and in many cases of proven vasculitis, it is possible to avoid systemic

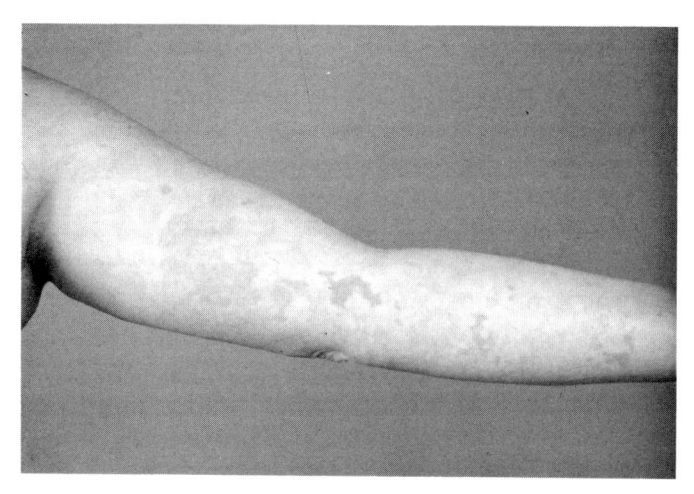

FIGURE 4.4 Urticaria in systemic lupus erythematosus

corticosteroid therapy[17]. Indomethacin, a prostaglandin inhibitor, has been reported to be of value in urticarial vasculitis, but it must be used with caution, as it has a similar effect to aspirin in those cases of chronic urticaria reacting to salicylates.

Physical urticaria

Dermographism

Wealing developing after scratch trauma occurs in about 5% of the normal population, a prevalence which is the same throughout all age groups. In these cases there is no itching, and it probably represents an increased physiological response in the skin. However, in addition to this, symptomatic dermographism, associated with large weals on scratch trauma, gives rise to paroxysms of itching. The condition may begin suddenly and last for a period of months or years. Passive transfer tests can be positive. Symptomatic dermographism characteristically develops in the young adult, although it may occur in childhood. Rarely it may follow acute urticaria, sometimes drug or parasite induced. Clinically it may be confused with chronic urticaria, but the weals of dermographism, although they may not be obviously scratch-provoked, last for only $\frac{1}{2}$–1 hour. Rubbing and pressure in these cases may cause larger swellings, and mimic angioedema, but they clear in a much shorter time, and of course the condition can readily be demonstrated by scratching the skin.

General dermographism (Figure 4.5) can occur in association with widespread insect bites, scabies, and following wasp and bee stings. The course of symptomatic dermographism is variable, but most cases settle down after a few years. Skin which has been repeatedly exposed to sunlight and weathering does not weal as readily as skin which remains covered, and sunbathing or ultraviolet light therapy is often helpful in management. H1 antagonists reduce the wealing tendency and usually continued treatment, which may be necessary for months or years, will keep the condition in check. As these patients are often young adults continuing with their jobs or study, the use of the non-sedating antihistamines has been of great value. The addition of H2 antagonists slightly increases the effect of the H1 antagonist, but this

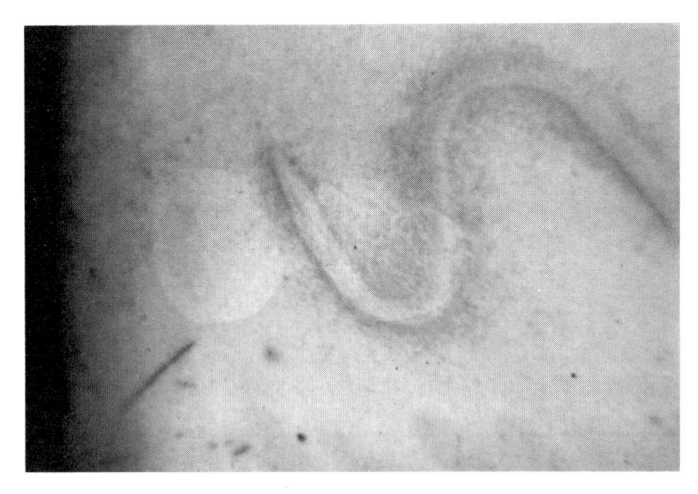

FIGURE 4.5 'S' for scabies. Dermographism in a patient with acarus infection

is not great enough to warrant the continued use of both drugs. Explanation and reassurance are important.

Other types of dermographism include:

1. Late dermographism – commences in 30–45 minutes and lasts 2–3 hours;
2. Delayed dermographism – commences 4–6 hours after a deep scratch and lasts 24 hours. Occurs in association with deep pressure urticaria;
3. Red dermographism – reaction to scratching or rubbing causing a red line with slight diffuse weal in some areas along it.

Cholinergic urticaria

Cholinergic urticaria occurs in response to exercise, general heat or emotional stress. Occasionally attacks follow spiced foods or alcoholic drinks. Although the incidence amongst other urticarial eruptions referred to hospital is from 5–7%, it is probably a very much commoner disorder in minor degrees. The average age of onset is about 15–16, but the condition can develop at an earlier age. The charac-

URTICARIA

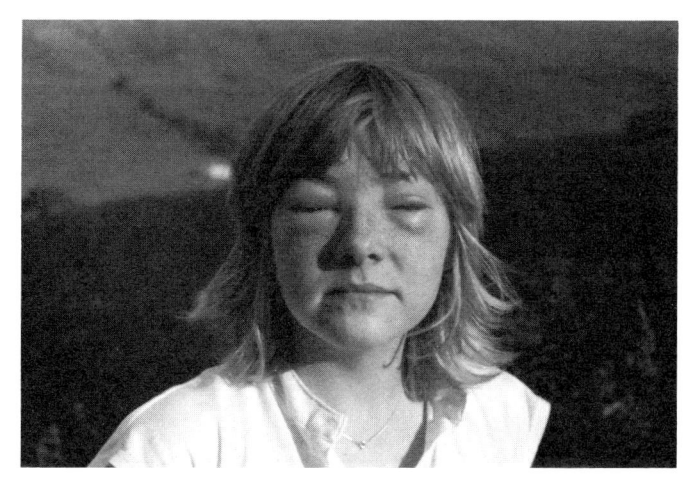

FIGURE 4.6 Cholinergic urticaria. Swelling of eyelids in severe attack

teristic weals are small, 2–3 mm in diameter, but in very severe cases they may merge together. The flare surrounding the weals is sometimes a prominent feature. Swelling of the face resembling angioedema[18] (Figure 4.6) and faintness and wheezing at the height of the eruption can occur.

The mechanism of the wealing is not fully understood, but the liberation of acetylcholine seems to play a part, eventually leading to histamine release. Attacks can be provoked by intracutaneous injections of methacholine chloride (mecholyl) 0.02% but easily the best clinical test for cholinergic urticaria is to exercise the patient in warm surroundings up to a point when there is profuse sweating. The test may be negative, particularly in those cases in which emotional factors seem to be the most important precipitating cause. As the weals last only $\frac{1}{2}$–1 hour the condition is readily differentiated from ordinary acute or chronic urticaria, but there may be confusion with other physical urticarias; for example, attacks of cholinergic urticaria due to exercise at the seaside could easily be confused with cold urticaria, dermographism or solar urticaria.

Cold urticaria

There are rare examples of urticaria secondary to cryoglobulinemia and other conditions, in which purpura and necrosis are usually associated with the cold-induced weals.

Familial cold urticaria, inherited as an autosomal dominant trait, is uncommon and becomes apparent shortly after birth or at an early age and is life long. On exposure to cold, particularly a chilling wind, the reaction begins after some 30 minutes and lasts up to 48 hours. The eruption, which occurs on exposed sites but sometimes elsewhere, consists of widespread erythematous patches and is associated with a burning sensation rather than itching. The mucous membranes are not involved and the condition is not precipitated by cold drinks. Fever, shivering attacks, arthralgia and headache occur. A neutrophil leucocytosis is usually present during attacks, and a neutrophil infiltrate on histology. Passive transfer tests are negative. Locally applied cold, such as the pressure of an ice cube, usually evokes no wealing.

Essential acquired cold urticaria, at any rate in minor degrees, is probably very much commoner than is indicated by the 2–3% of patients presenting with urticaria in hospital. Although commoner in cold climates and in winter months, it may occur in tropical countries, as the main stimulus of the urticaria is a drop in the temperature. It occurs at any age but is commoner in the young adult[19]. It may begin after some incident, such as a severe sting, an infection or a drug eruption.

After exposure of an area of skin to a drop in temperature, a weal develops on rewarming. The weal itches, and then clears after a quarter to one hour, and leaves normal skin, although minor purpura occasionally develops at the site of maximum wealing. The commonest precipitating events are cold winds, immersion in cold water, or contact with cold surfaces, usually for a few minutes. Evaporation of sweat, or wet skin from rain, may lead to wealing. Swelling of the mouth, tongue and pharynx and even attacks of abdominal pain may very rarely be induced by very cold foods or iced drinks.

If the wealing is widespread and severe, syncope may occur and loss of consciousness has occasionally been responsible for deaths from drowning. The usual way of testing for cold urticaria is to apply an ice cube for 5–10 minutes to the patient's skin and weals appear when the skin is rewarmed. Another test commonly used is to immerse the arm in a basin of cold tap water for 10 minutes and when removed localized or diffuse wealing is apparent. In many cases the condition improves over a period of months or years. The mechanism is not fully understood. Histamine undoubtedly plays a part. Passive transfer has been demonstrated with serum of affected patients. The factor is probably an IgE immunoglobulin, and, as with dermographism, the physical stimulus presumably releases the responsible antigen.

There is really no satisfactory treatment. Some cases have improved after so-called desensitization by exposure to cold water, gradually increasing the time of exposure and decreasing the temperature of the water, but many patients find this technique difficult and distressing. Antihistamines reduce the wealing and may help some severe cases. They may also be of value if taken 2–3 hours before an expected exposure. At one time the antihistamine cyproheptadine was commonly used in cold urticaria but terfenadine and astemizole probably have as much effect and can be given in larger doses if necessary. Doxepin, a tricyclic anti-depressant with antihistamine properties has also been used. Doxantrazole, a mast cell stabilizing drug, helped in a series of patients, but it has not become a regular therapy for cold urticaria.

Other physical urticarias

Mixtures of dermographism, cholinergic urticaria and cold urticaria occur[19]. Other patterns of cold urticaria, direct heat and vibratory urticaria have been described. Solar urticaria is a well-recognized but rare condition. The weals develop a few minutes after exposure and clear in $\frac{1}{2}$–1 hour after exposure has ceased. There are different types depending on particular wave lengths which are usually in the ultra-violet range. The timing and lack of scaling readily distinguish this condition from actinic dermatitis and prurigo.

Cholinergic urticaria, cold urticaria and dermographism may all be worsened after contact with water of different temperatures. There is, in addition, the rare condition of aquagenic urticaria when small papules develop at the site of contact with water[20]. The mechanism of this condition is not understood but the diagnosis should only be accepted if the typical weals occur on application of a compress of water applied for some 30 minutes and preferably kept at body heat. Aquagenic urticaria has to be distinguished from the more common aquagenic pruritus in which there is itching but no weals[21].

Deep pressure urticaria

Pressure urticaria is characterized by the development of deep swellings, often painful, in the skin and subcutaneous tissue, 4–8 hours after pressure has been applied to the skin and they last for 12–48 hours. Any skin site may be involved; for example, the soles of the feet after walking or standing with pressure on one particular site, as on a ladder; the palms may be affected after clapping, or pressure from a tool; and the shoulders, trunk and limbs after leaning against a hard edge for some minutes (Figure 4.7). In view of the long latent period before the weals develop, the patients may not readily associate the swellings with such pressure, because immediately afterwards the skin looks quite normal. If there are numerous swellings, general malaise, aching and headaches may develop.

One diagnostic problem arises because at least 50% of the patients

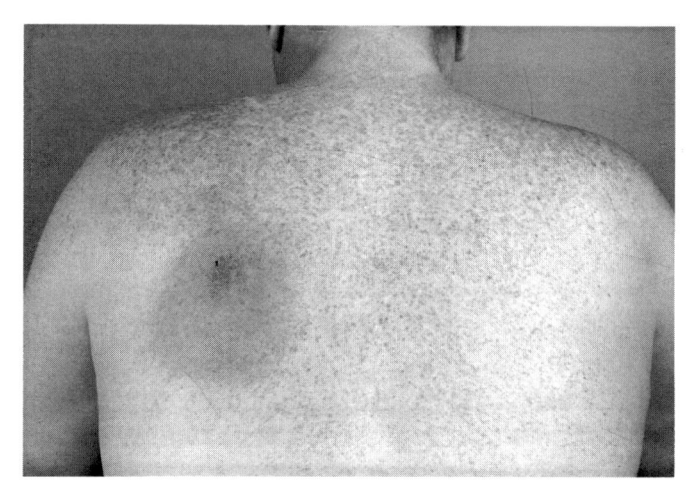

FIGURE 4.7 Deep pressure urticaria after leaning back against a hard chair

showing true pressure urticaria also have chronic urticarial weals. There is a further confusion in relation to weals at pressure sites, because in ordinary chronic urticaria, weals may be more apparent where there has been pressure against the skin, for example where there has been tight clothing (Köbner weals) (Figure 4.8). However these develop at the height of the general urticarial eruption and fade as the general weals clear distinguishing them from true pressure urticaria.

Pressure urticaria occurs with different degrees of severity and may be a minor nuisance or so severe that it requires a change of occupation or markedly limits social activities. It lasts many years but most cases gradually improve with time. Various methods of testing have been used but basically consist of hanging weights over the arms, shoulders or legs. A common test is to use a 7–14 kilogram weight, which is suspended by stuffed stockinette and left over the arm or shoulder for 5–10 minutes. However this is quite often negative, as the causative pressure is of a shearing nature and a good testing procedure has yet to be introduced.

The nature of pressure urticaria has not been finally determined. Histologically there is an infiltration with eosinophils, and sometimes neutrophils, with endothelial thickening of the capillaries.

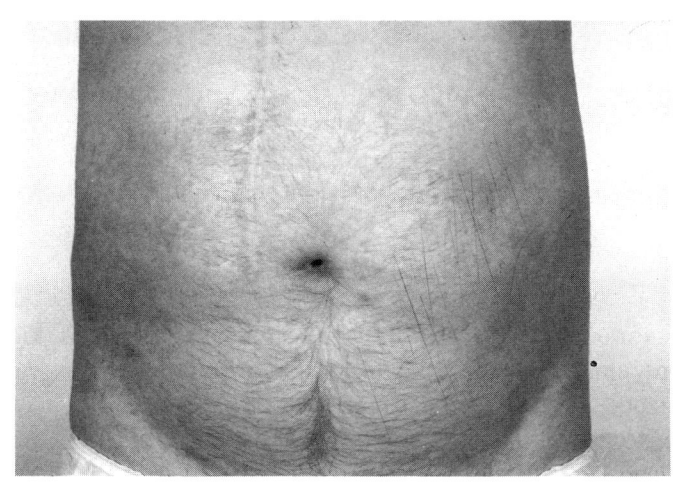

FIGURE 4.8 Chronic urticaria – weal at the site of pressure from clothing (Köbner weal)

Immunofluorescent studies are negative. The mediators involved are unknown but kinin release has been suggested[22].

Antihistamines, even in large doses, do not have any apparent clinical effect, although these may help any associated chronic urticaria. Systemic corticosteroids will control the condition but are rarely used as it is necessary to give standard doses for a long time and there are often problems with side-effects. If patients are subjected to a lot of skin pressure which they know from previous experience is going to cause a severe attack, they can reduce the severity by immediately taking a large dose of prednisolone, tapered off in the next 24 hours. It has been suggested that tranexamic acid, as used in hereditary angioedema, helps in deep pressure urticaria but results with this drug seem to vary and it is far from regular in its effect.

Hereditary angioedema

Hereditary angioedema (HAE) is a genetic disease due to deficiency of C1 inhibitor. Ordinary angioedema is a common component of urticaria and occurs in association with urticaria or on its own (see earlier). Ordinary angioedema may be familial but this must be distinguished from HAE which has a specific biochemistry.

The disease is inherited as a simple autosomal dominant and usually starts in late childhood. It is caused by a deficiency of a neuraminoglycoprotein produced in the liver. In patients with HAE the inhibitor is usually reduced to about 20% but in a variant form it is present in normal quantities but with a deficient activity[23]. Either form can be recognized quite easily in specially equipped laboratories and affected individuals with either form tend to have extremely low C4 and C2 levels most of their life.

There is sometimes a prodromal rash before the main attacks and this consists of a few or sometimes many lesions scattered chiefly over the trunk. They are annular or figurate in outline and the spreading edge slightly wealed.

The swellings often arise spontaneously (Figure 4.9) but may occur at the site of trauma such as a blow or perhaps dental trauma. They are usually single swellings but sometimes three or four may be present at one time. The lesions may be slightly painful. The danger is oedema

URTICARIA

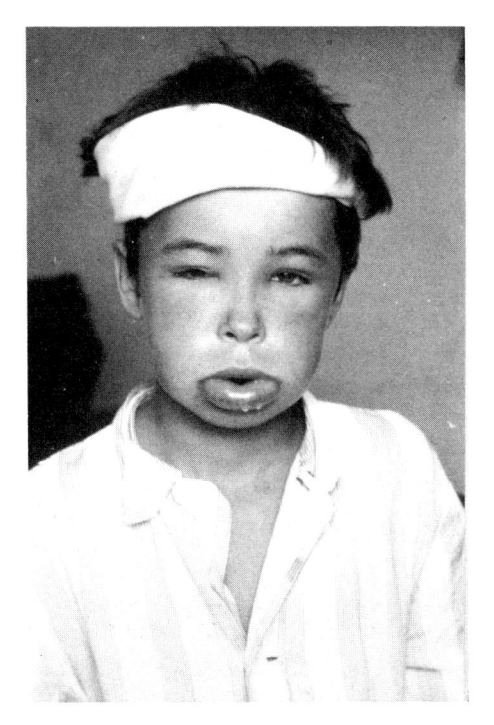

FIGURE 4.9 Hereditary angioedema. Handkerchief on the head ready to cover his face when in public

of the larynx, pharynx, trachea and bronchi which may lead to respiratory obstruction and asphyxia. It is the spread of oedema down the bronchi which makes the condition so difficult to treat and even tracheostomy may be ineffective. The mortality varies from family to family but in some families 25% of the members have died of respiratory obstruction by late adult life.

Some patients have in addition to, or instead of, subcutaneous swellings, attacks of abdominal pain due to bowel oedema. The pain is often severe and colicky and there may be diarrhoea. The bowel oedema can be diagnosed on a follow-through barium meal by the 'stacked coin' or 'picket fence' appearance. These patients with recurrent abdominal pain are very often misdiagnosed[24].

It has been known for 25 years that methyl testosterone improves patients with HAE but this has a virilizing activity and in the last 5 years danazol 200–800 mg daily or stanozolol 2.5–5.0 mg daily have been used as they are able to increase the production of the C1 inhibitor without serious side-effects. The level of C1 inhibitor with such treatment can return to normal but in many cases a smaller dose will control clinical symptoms[25]. In children there must be worries about the effects on growth and sexual characters but experience over the last few years has been reassuring. Patients who have had severe attacks are now kept trouble-free by the continued administration of these drugs. They have largely taken the place of epsilon amino caproic acid or its derivative, tranexamic acid, which inhibit the activation of plasmin from plasminogen and thus have a sparing effect on the C1 inhibitor. Tranexamic acid can be used in conjunction with anabolic steroids.

If acute attacks occur in patients who are inadequately controlled, or in undiagnosed cases, the urgent treatment is by infusion of fresh frozen plasma. However the purified preparation of C1 inhibitor, free of C4, is now available and has taken over from the fresh frozen plasma. The preparation is expensive but has a shelf life of 1–2 years and can be kept in a domestic refrigerator. It can, therefore, be held by the patient or the doctor at the centre where the patient would report to for immediate treatment if necessary.

There is a rare non-hereditary form of angioedema due to deficiency of C1 inhibitor[26]. Many of these patients have abnormal B-cell proliferations, for example, lymphosarcoma, and there is a consumption of the C1 inhibitor, but low C1 levels are found in the serum.

Most patients with HAE suffer only from their angioedema but some 2–5% develop a variety of immune complex diseases, of which systemic lupus erythematosus is the commonest.

REFERENCES

1. Warin, R. P. and Champion, R. H. (1974). *Urticaria.* pp. 33–73 (London: W. B. Saunders)
2. Boonk, W. J. and van Ketel, W. G. (1982). The role of penicillin in the pathogenesis of chronic urticaria. *Br. J. Dermatol.*, **106,** 183–90
3. James, J. and Warin, R. P. (1971). An assessment of the role of Candida albicans and food yeasts in chronic urticaria. *Br. J. Dermatol.*, **84,** 227–37

4. James, J. and Warin, R. P. (1970). Chronic urticaria: the effect of aspirin. *Br. J. Dermatol.*, **82**, 204
5. Juhlin, L. (1985). Food additives in urticaria. In Champion, R. H., Greaves, M. W., Kobza Black, A. and Pye, R. J. *The Urticarias*, Chap. 13 (Edinburgh: Churchill Livingstone)
6. Michaelsson, G. and Juhlin, L. (1973). Urticaria induced by preservatives and dye additives in foods and drugs. *Br. J. Dermatol.*, **88**, 525–32
7. Warin, R. P. and Smith, R. J. (1982). Role of tartrazine in chronic urticaria. *Br. Med. J.*, **284**, 1443–4
8. Matthews, C., Boss, J. M., Warin, R. P. *et al.* (1979). The effect of H1 and H2 histamine antagonists on symptomatic dermographism. *Br. J. Dermatol.*, **101**, 57–61
9. Commens, C. A. and Greaves, M. W. (1978). Cimetidine in chronic idiopathic urticaria: A randomized double-blind study. *Br. J. Dermatol.*, **99**, 675–9
10. Monroe, E. W., Cohen, S. H., Kalbfleisch, J. *et al.* (1981). Combined H1 and H2 antihistamine therapy in chronic urticaria. *Arch. Dermatol.*, **117**, 404–7
11. Saihan, E. M. (1981). Ketotifen and terbutaline in urticaria. *Br. J. Dermatol.*, **104**, 205–6
12. Champion, R. H., Roberts, S. O. B., Carpenter, R. G. and Roger, J. H. (1969). Urticaria and angio-edema: a review of 554 cases. *Br. J. Dermatol.*, **81**, 588–97
13. Gleich, G. J., Schroeter, Al., Marcoux, P., Sachs, M. J., O'Connell, E. J. and Kohler, P. F. (1984). Episodic angioedema associated with eosinophilia. *New Engl. J. Med.*, **310**, 1621–6
14. Monroe, E. W., Schulz, C. I., Maize, J. C. and Jordon, R. E. (1981). Vasculitis in chronic urticaria: an immunopathologic study. *J. Invest. Dermatol.*, **76**, 103–7
15. Russell Jones, R., Bhogal, B., Dash, A. and Schiffereli, J. (1983). Urticaria and vasculitis: a continuum of histopathological and immunopathological changes. *Br. J. Dermatol.*, **108**, 695–703
16. Soter, N. A., Austen, K. F. and Gigli, I. (1974). Urticaria and arthralgias as manifestations of necrotizing angiitis (vasculitis). *J. Invest. Dermatol.*, **63**, 485–90
17. Warin, R. P. (1983). Urticarial vasculitis. *Br. Med. J.*, **286**, 1919–20
18. Lawrence, C. M., Jorizzo, J. L., Kobza Black, A., Coutts, A. and Greaves, M. W. (1981). Cholinergic urticaria with associated angio-oedema. *Br. J. Dermatol.*, **105**, 543–50
19. Neittaanmaki, H. (1985). Cold urticaria. Clinical findings in 220 patients. *J. Am. Acad. Dermatol.*, **13**, 636–43
20. Illig, L., Paul, E., Bruck, K., Schwennicke, E. H. P. (1980). Experimental investigations on the trigger mechanism of the generalized type of heat and cold urticaria by means of a climatic chamber. *Acta Dermato-Venereol.*, **60**, 373–80
21. Greaves, M. W., Black, A. K., Eady, R. A. J. and Coutts, A. (1981). Aquagenic pruritus. *Br. Med. J.*, **282**, 2008–11
22. Winkelmann, R. K., Wilhelmj, C. M. and Horner, F. A. (1965). Experimental studies on dermographism. *Arch. Dermatol.*, **92**, 436–40
23. Lachmann, P. J. (1985). Hereditary angio-oedema. In Champion, R. H., Greaves, M. W., Kobza Black, A. and Pye, R. J. *The Urticarias* Chap. 25. (Edinburgh: Churchill Livingstone)
24. Warin, R. P. and Higgs, E. R. (1982). Acute and recurrent abdominal pain due to angio-oedema. *Br. Med. J.*, **284**, 1912

25. Warin, A. P., Greaves, M. W., Gatecliff, M., Williamson, D. M. and Warin, R. P. (1980). Treatment of hereditary angio-oedema by low dose attenuated androgens: disassociation of clinical response from levels of C_1 esterase inhibitor and C_4. *Br. J. Dermatol.*, **103,** 405–9
26. Caldwell, J. R., Ruddy, S., Schur, P. H. and Austen, K. F. (1972). Acquired C1 inhibitor deficiency in lymphosarcoma. *Clin. Immunol. Immunopathol.*, **1,** 39–52

5
PSORIASIS

T. C. HINDSON

DEFINITION

Psoriasis is a common skin disorder usually consisting of sharply-defined raised plaques with a distinctive colour varying from salmon pink to dull red. Each lesion is topped with characteristic silvery scales.

The condition is genetically determined and frequently runs a long but unpredictable course in which the patient's general health is usually unaffected. There are several atypical forms and there is sometimes an associated arthritis.

PREVALENCE

It has been estimated that the condition afflicts approximately 2% of the adult population of North West Europe and that men are more frequently affected than women[1]. It is rare in American Indians and in Africans, particularly in Nigeria[2].

The incidence is increased in isolated communities where inter-marriage has taken place such as the Faroe islands and mining communities in North East England (own unpublished data).

AETIOLOGY

The aetiology still remains obscure and although advances have been made in many fields which will now be discussed, the abnormal results recorded still do not solve the 'chicken and egg' question. Are they the cause or the result of the disease process?

Genetics

Unequivocal evidence exists to support a genetic predisposition and there are several well-documented studies of identical twins. Several family studies were summarized by Marcusson *et al.*[3] and they suggested that there was a 'predisposing' gene for psoriasis on chromosome No 6 near the HLA region.

Biochemistry

Psoriasis is characterized by greatly increased epidermal cell production and turnover and most biochemical studies of enzymes in the skin merely reflect this increased activity with a shift from the oxidative to glycolytic metabolic pathway.

Blood biochemistry is usually normal. In long-standing extensive psoriasis deficiency of serum B12 and red cell folate may arise. In the rare form of acute fulminating pustular psoriasis, acute electrolyte disturbances occur with diminution of plasma volume and protein.

Recently Camp *et al.*[4] have shown that intradermal injection of leukotrienes can produce microabscesses with a histological appearance very similar to that of developing psoriasis.

Further evidence to support the role of leukotrienes in the aetiology of psoriasis was provided by Allen and Littlewood[5] who reported the favourable response of psoriasis to therapy with benoxaprofen, a drug which blocked the enzymic pathway of leukotriene synthesis. This drug has now been withdrawn because of other serious side-effects.

Trauma

Psoriasis is frequently exacerbated following major trauma, surgical operations and childbirth. Local injuries to the skin such as cuts, burns, or other skin infection frequently lead later to localized psoriasis at the site of injury (Köbner phenomenon).

Stress and psychogenic factors

These are difficult to quantify but most clinical dermatologists accept that they play a definite provocative role. A bereavement, sudden redundancy, unhappiness at work, at home or school all play a part. Seville[6] published data attributing stress as a major aetiological agent.

Infection

Streptococcal and upper respiratory tract viral infections frequently precipitate an attack of psoriasis, usually of the guttate type, and it is often the first manifestation of the disease in younger patients.

Warmth and sunlight

Psoriasis tends to improve in sunny conditions although sunburn can precipitate psoriasis in the affected areas.

Drugs

Withdrawal of systemic steroid therapy may be followed by an exacerbation of psoriasis and many dermatologists believe that the increased incidence of severe psoriasis may be due to prior injudicious use of topical steroids. Antimalarials may provoke generalized exfoliative erythroderma in existing psoriasis.

Of particular interest is the effect of lithium salts, now used to treat affective psychoses. These cause an increase in the numbers of circulating polymorphs and will produce a dose-related provocation of the complaint in known psoriatics[7]. This drug suggests itself as a further tool for the investigation of the aetiology of psoriasis.

Immunology

An immunological aetiology for psoriasis has been proposed and increased numbers of 'T' helper cell lymphocytes have been demonstrated in active lesions and a decreased number of total lymphocytes with relative predominance of 'T' suppressor cells in receding lesions.

PATHOLOGY

The earliest histological change is invasion of the epidermis by polymorphs and small micro abscesses, known as Munro abscesses, form in the lower epidermis. The whole epidermis shows increased activity and immature keratinocytes reach the surface still retaining their nuclei (parakeratosis). The epidermis becomes thickened and folded to accommodate its increased volume and capillaries in the dermal papillae are dilated.

MODE OF ONSET

Psoriasis is uncommon before the age of 3 but may appear for the first time at any time in life. However its first appearance is usually in the mid-twenties with females tending to be affected at a younger age.

CLINICAL TYPES

Plaque psoriasis

This is the commonest variety (Figures 5.1 and 5.2). Plaque size may vary from a few millimetres to many centimetres. Any area of the

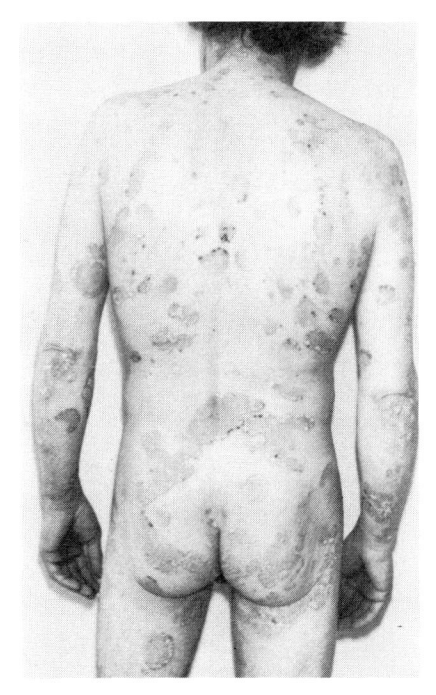

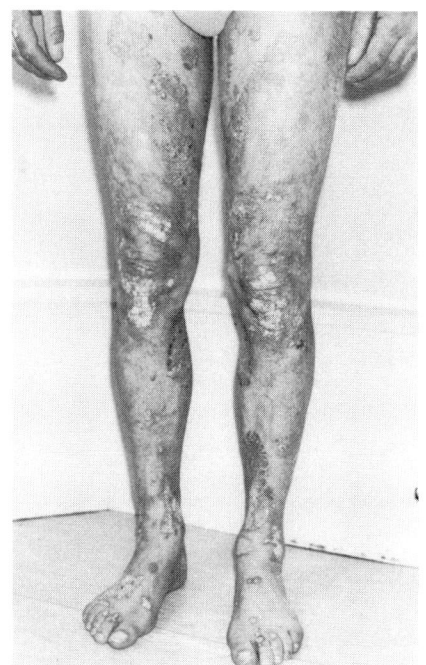

FIGURES 5.1 and 5.2 Chronic plaque psoriasis

body may be affected although the face is usually spared. The knees, elbows and scalp are the commonest areas affected. Here the lesions show the classical silvery scales which continue to be shed in abundance while the lesions are active, to the extent that the patient may need to vacuum clean his house daily.

Plaque psoriasis is modified by the affected site. Lesions of the intertriginous skin tend to be moist and exudative and not scaly.

Lesions of the scalp (Figure 5.3) tend to show only thick white scales and sometimes appear to be climbing up the hair shafts (pityriasis amiantacea) with a boggy appearance of the underlying scalp.

Palmar lesions are thinner than elsewhere but still in small discs with scales. Gentle removal of the scale will reveal multiple small bleeding capillaries which is a useful diagnostic sign to differentiate it from other disorders such as ringworm and eczema.

On the penis there is frequently only a small discoid lesion on the tip and sometimes this may be the only lesion on the body in which

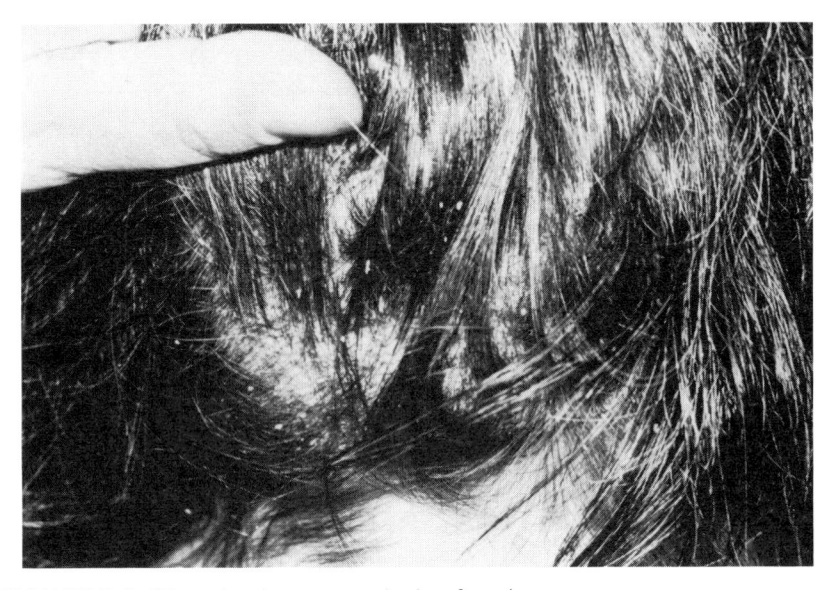

FIGURE 5.3 Chronic plaque psoriasis of scalp

case removal of the scale as described above is also a useful diagnostic aid.

Psoriasis of the nails

This frequently occurs in association with plaque psoriasis but may be the only manifestation of the disease. The nail has only a limited number of ways in which it can react to inflammatory skin disorders so that the changes seen may occur in other disorders such as eczema and lichen planus.

Pitting – multiple small pit marks appear and nails of both hands and feet may be affected. The lesions usually affect the nails of both limbs in a symmetrical fashion and are not often seen in other skin disorders.

Hyperkeratosis – here there is a thickening of the nail plate, ridging and cracking. Lesions due to psoriasis tend to be symmetrical but are not diagnostic and samples must be examined to exclude ringworm. This also applies to patients with psoriasis elsewhere on the body particularly if topical steroid therapy has been previously used.

PSORIASIS

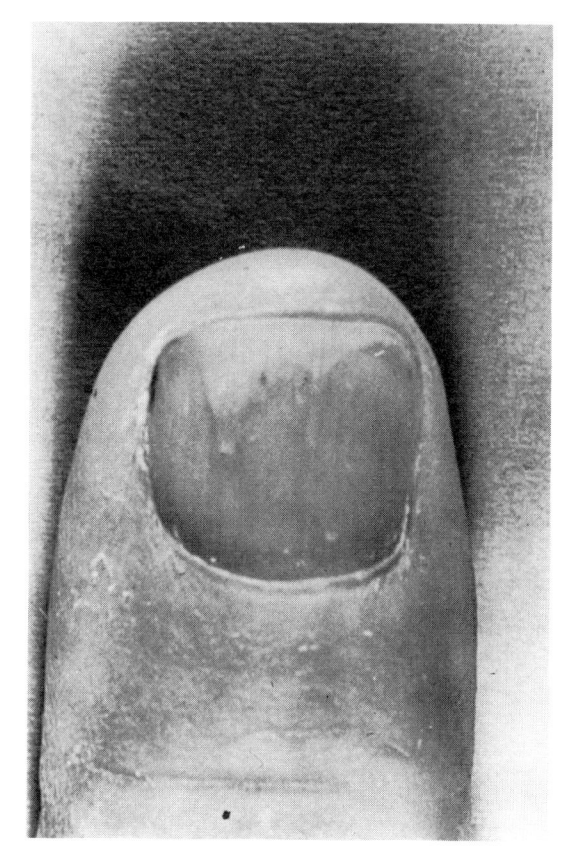

FIGURE 5.4 Nail psoriasis illustrating onycholysis

Onycholysis (Figure 5.4) – this describes the change seen where the nail separates from the nail bed so that a white area like the terminal part of the nail spreads backwards towards the nail base. The onset is often rapid and the underlying area may become infected with a mixture of fungi and bacteria giving a greeny brown discolouration and sometimes a foul smell.

Nail psoriasis of all types is frequently seen in association with a psoriatic arthritis of the distal interphalangeal joints (Figure 5.5).

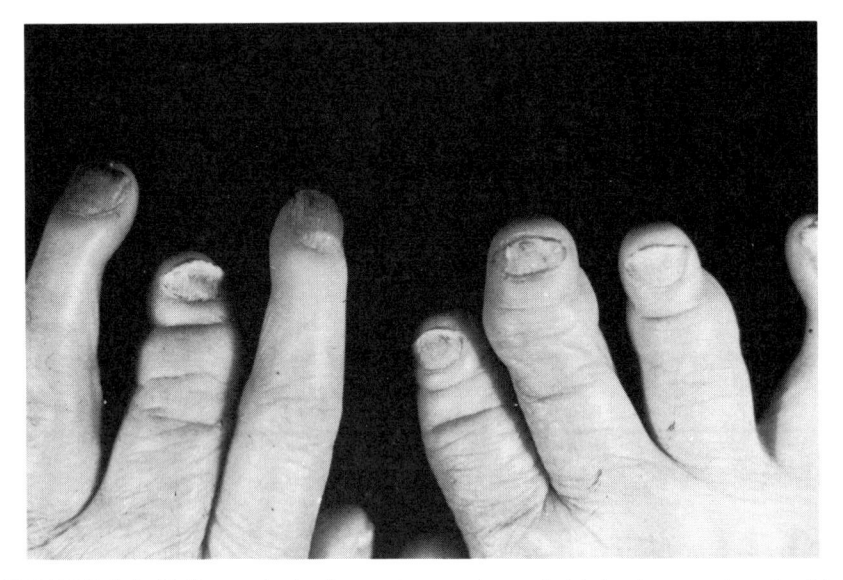

FIGURE 5.5 Nail psoriasis (hyperkeratosis and ridging) associated with psoriatic arthritis

Guttate psoriasis

This derives its name from Latin (*gutta*: a drop). The lesions are small and multiple. The onset is sudden and the whole body may be covered rapidly.

This type frequently follows upper respiratory infections particularly streptococcal. Frequently it is the first manifestation of the disease so that younger patients tend to be affected. Physical health is unaffected but the patients are understandably alarmed.

Erythrodermic psoriasis

Generalized and sudden erythroderma may involve the whole body and may be the first manifestation of the disease. More usually it evolves from chronic plaque psoriasis where treatment with topical agents has been applied in too strong concentrations.

The gross increase in skin blood flow may result in hypothermia and in longer-standing cases diminution of plasma protein and sometimes onset of left ventricular failure. Hypothermia is manifest initially with shivering, and measurement of rectal temperature, which gives a more accurate picture of body core temperature, may be normal. All over application of a dilute fluorinated steroid ointment with stockinette dressings will usually reverse these early changes.

Pustular psoriasis

There are several forms of this in which small pustules appear either on pre-existing plaques or *de novo* on normal skin. Generalized pustular psoriasis (Von Zumbusch) may be life-threatening and treatment is urgently required. Accordingly these types will be discussed in the section dealing with treatment later.

Pustular psoriasis of palms and soles

This condition otherwise known as palmo-plantar pustulosis (PPP) consists of sterile itchy pustules on an erythemato-squamous background affecting the palms and soles. Frequently palms or soles alone are involved. Psoriasis may be present elsewhere on the body but more usually is absent. The lesions tend to be symmetrical on both limbs and it is important to exclude ringworm infection, which may mimic the condition, by taking samples of blister epidermis for microscopic examination after preparation of the sample in potassium hydroxide.

Keratoderma blenorrhagicum

This is a variety of palmo-plantar pustulosis which occurs in about 10% of cases suffering from Reiter's syndrome (arthritis and uveitis in association with non-specific urethritis or gonorrhoea).

Topical therapy as outlined later for PPP is usually adequate but where arthritis is also severe, a course of methotrexate over 2 months is an excellent therapy for both conditions.

Psoriasis arthritis

This arthritis affects about 7% of patients with psoriasis and may resemble rheumatoid arthritis but Rose–Waaler and other rheumatoid serum tests are negative.

Onset is usually more insidious than rheumatoid and it may frequently remain monoarticular.

A common variety affects the distal interphalangeal joints of the fingers in which case psoriatic nail changes are also present. X-rays show bone resorption of the terminal phalanges, the name 'drawing pin' phalanx being given to the picture.

A more aggressive form, arthritis mutilans, may affect the hands with a strong resemblance to rheumatoid arthritis, resulting in gross bone resorption, joint destruction, subluxation and permanent deformity (Figure 5.6).

Psoriasis with other skin disorders

The clinician must be vigilant for conditions which have damaged the skin and in which psoriasis has arisen as a Köbner phenomenon. Scabies, contact eczema (particularly from nickel), ringworm and impetigo are common examples. These conditions should receive appropriate therapy before attention is directed at the psoriasis.

TREATMENT OF PSORIASIS

Assessment

It is important to make an overall assessment of the patient and why he or she has presented for treatment at this particular time. Generalized guttate psoriasis, though not affecting the patient's physical health, is a cause for acute alarm with its sudden dramatic appear-

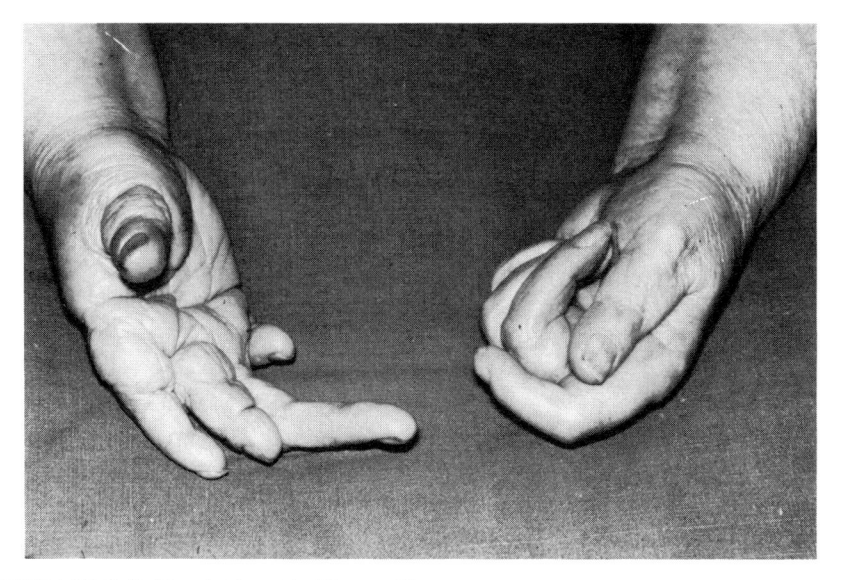

FIGURE 5.6 Psoriatic arthritis mutilans

ance and the patient may have to undress in the view of others such as at school, or communal works baths as at coal mines.

Many patients may tolerate limited plaque psoriasis, particularly of elbows and knees, for years and are only referred because the lesions are discovered at a routine medical examination, perhaps for insurance purposes. The patient may still not wish to have any treatment or will not bother to use a prescription.

Assessment of the patients socio-economic background and intelligence is important to ascertain whether the patient has the home facilities or sufficient intelligence to cope with topical therapies, many of which are difficult and messy to use. Patients living alone may not be able to treat areas on the back or apply dressings.

Time spent in sympathetic explanation is not wasted and may save future unnecessary consultations.

It is also important to assess motivation, as to how keen the patient is to have the disease cleared. Where in-patient facilities permit it is a good idea to admit the patient with plaque psoriasis arising for the first time, so that he can see how treatment is carried out and meet other psoriatics under therapy to see how common the condition is and also enable him to carry out similar therapy on his own at home in the event of recurrence.

In any case the patient should not be allowed to leave the department without having had a further explanation and practical demonstration of topical applications by skilled nursing staff, in addition to that already given by the physician. Other causes of motivation should lurk at the back of the mind, particularly medico-legal: is the patient going to use the complaint as part of grounds for divorce, or as a basis for a claim for industrial dermatitis?

General measures

If the patient is otherwise in good health there is no doubt that the old-fashioned remedy of rest is a good one. A sunny seaside holiday may do much more for the condition than many medications. Alternatively a period of in-patient therapy may relieve the patient and his family from the difficulties of home treatment and in itself provide a period of rest. Mild sedatives may be necessary initially but patients who are depressed because of their disease rarely need antidepressant drugs, as depression rapidly lifts when the patients can see improvement as a result of therapy and explanation.

Patients who are genuinely suicidal are rarely so because of psoriasis alone and psychiatric assistance should be obtained urgently.

Diet plays no part in the management of this condition. However, if the patient is so convinced that a particular foodstuff improves the condition then this should not be discouraged, provided it is known not to be injurious to health in other ways. Some patients wish to attend faith healers, psychotherapists or visit special spa baths and similarly this should not be discouraged provided the patient is not being financially overburdened by such measures. Placebo therapy can be very effective. Patients with acute generalized pustular psoriasis should always be admitted as soon as possible for in-patient therapy and rest.

Topical therapy

As a general rule acute eruptive psoriatic lesions should be treated with bland applications initially. Liberal applications of zinc cream with overall tube gauze dressings are very effective. In our own unit (unpublished observations) we have found a more preferable application is a cream containing peanut oil 25% in equal parts of ung. emuls. aquosum and soft paraffin. These applications can be given for a few days until more powerful agents are introduced.

Dithranol (Anthralin USA)

This has become the standard topical therapeutic regimen for most cases of plaque psoriasis in dermatological units in the United Kingdom and has in fact been in use for over 70 years. It has the unfortunate drawback that it produces unpleasant brown staining on all clothing and sheets which appears when the articles are washed and is then irremovable. It must be introduced at low concentrations and increases in strength must be carefully judged to avoid burning the patient. Although the substance has been in use for many years its popularity was greatly increased when Ingram outlined his own procedures for its use in 1953[8].

The Ingram regime

This regime is still very popular in many centres and can be carried out as a daily outpatient procedure. The regimen is as follows:

(1) The patient takes a bath (90 l) to which 120 ml of alcoholic extract of coal tar has been added. Ingram stated that the object of this is to sensitize the lesions to ultraviolet light.

(2) The patient then receives a dose of UVB radiation building up gradually to a sub-erythema level. Ingram introduced this because sunlight was beneficial for psoriasis[8].

(3) Dithranol 0.05% in stiffened Lassars Paste with 2% salicylic acid (to prevent oxidation of dithranol) is then carefully applied exactly to each lesion with care taken to avoid contact with normal

skin. According to progress the strength of dithranol is gradually increased to 0.5% and in some cases 1%.

When the application is completed the lesions are powdered with talcum and all the affected parts covered with a stockinette dressing. The patient can then dress and go about his daily work although dithranol does tend to penetrate the stockinette towards the end of 24 hours.

Clearance times of approximately 3 weeks are claimed for this technique. Seville (1975)[9] found however, that clearance times were of a similar order if dithranol alone was used without tar baths and UVB.

Modifications of dithranol therapy

(1) *Short contact (minutes) therapy:* Runne and Kunze[10] introduced the concept of applying high concentrations of dithranol for very short periods working up from 10 minutes to 1 hour, after which the ointment is washed off, making this a very suitable outpatient therapy. However, burning, particularly with high concentrations of dithranol has been found to be a significant problem[11].

(2) *Short contact dithranol plus UVA (DUVA):* In 1982 Hindson *et al.*[12] noted that dithranol is photoactive and that its absorption spectrum is almost the mirror image of the emission spectrum of UVA lamps used in most PUVA units with peak absorption and emission respectively at approximately 360 nm. Over 400 cases have been treated in our unit since then. There is debate as to what part UVA radiation plays but we have shown that UVA reduced burning on normal skin to which dithranol has been previously applied.

The regime is as follows: dithranol 0.1% in soft paraffin plus 2% salicylic acid is applied to all lesions. Exact application to the lesions does not appear to matter greatly. The patient then wears a disposable theatre gown for one hour, and then the dithranol is wiped off with a tissue and the patient takes a bath to which has been added an anionic detergent (TeePol) and an emollient; Alpha Keri (Bristol Myers), Balneum (Merck Ltd) and Oilatum (Stiefel Laboratories) have all been found satisfactory.

The patient then receives 20 J UVA in a standard PUVA cabinet. If the patient complains of dryness of the skin a liberal supply of emollient cream is given (ung. emuls. aquosum or unguentum Merck).

After 4 days dithranol concentration is increased to 1% and after a further 3 or 4 days to 3% and after a similar interval, if necessary, to 5%.

The median clearance time with this regimen is 15 days. We have found it particularly useful for clearance of acute guttate psoriasis in which 0.1% dithranol is used and applied all over including normal skin. Clearance times for this type of psoriasis have been in the order of 10 days.

We have used similar concentrations of dithranol at similar intervals without UVA on outpatients and although clearance times are somewhat longer results have been good. Two points of detail must be stressed to the patient who is using home treatment:

(a) Wear plastic gloves to avoid dithranol staining of nails when applying medication.

(b) Staining of the bath occurs particularly with high concentrations of dithranol. This should be removed immediately with a bleach solution Vortex (Procter & Gamble Ltd), or Domestos (Lever Bros). Failure to remove the stain immediately will result in a permanent mark on the bath.

Tar and UVB radiation

Goeckerman in 1925 introduced a regimen using crude coal tar and ultraviolet light for the treatment of psoriasis with good results. Crude coal tar is exceptionally messy to use and becoming more difficult to obtain as gas works cease production in the United Kingdom.

Several cosmetically acceptable tar gels are now available and can be used on an out-patient basis.

A recent American study[13] reported excellent results using a purified tar gel equivalent to 5% crude coal tar combined with a mixture of UVA and UVB radiation. After 1 week of in-patient therapy they were able to continue treatment on an out-patient basis and record a clearing time of 3 weeks followed by maintenance therapy of diminishing frequency over 2–3 months.

Topical steroids

Most dermatologists have abandoned the use of whole body application of topical steroids because of their well-known systemic side-effects and also because cessation of therapy usually leads to a fairly quick relapse usually worse than the initial presentation.

They are however still useful as whole body applications over a period of days to calm down an acute attack prior to the use of some other modality such as PUVA (see below).

Moderately potent steroids are probably still the treatment of choice for psoriasis in intertriginous areas and around the ears.

Psoriasis of the scalp

Mild lesions may respond to a proprietary tar shampoo alone, of which several are available. More scaly lesions respond to a weak steroid and tar cream (Alphosyl HC (Stafford Miller)) applied at night before the morning tar shampoo.

Thick crusted lesions respond well to a 0.1% dithranol plus 17% urea cream (Psoradrate 0.1% (Norwich Eaton)) applied at night. The patient is provided with a disposable paper cap to prevent staining of bed linen and the normal tar shampoo is performed in the morning.

A topical steroid in gel base (Synalar Gel (ICI)) is useful for treating acute exudative lesions.

In our experience alcoholic solutions of steroids labelled as 'scalp lotions' are of no value in the treatment of scalp psoriasis.

Psoralen plus UVA radiation (PUVA therapy)

This involves the taking orally of 8-methoxy psoralen followed 2 hours later by UVA radiation. It constitutes one of the major advances in the treatment of psoriasis and was introduced in the United Kingdom in 1977 and now most centres are able to offer this facility. It has the major advantage that the drug is non-toxic and the treatment does not involve the use of messy ointments.

Great care must be exercised in the initial stages of therapy to ensure accurate measurement of the UVA dosage. Initial radiation doses are related to the patient's skin colour and dosage of psoralen according to the patient's weight[14]. The long-term effects of this treatment are not yet known but definite skin changes akin to solar damage occur in long-term therapy which include lentigines, keratoses, elastosis and a few recorded cases of basal cell carcinomata. In the latter group the association is difficult to prove.

Because of these side-effects most dermatologists have confined the treatment to patients over the age of 45 who have had multiple admissions for topical therapy or in younger patients for limited treatment periods or for those whose psoriasis has been so severe as to warrant therapy with antimetabolites such as methotrexate (see below).

In our department we regard it as a maintenance therapy, having first cleared patients initially with topical therapy. Some patients only attend once monthly for PUVA therapy and one should not always aim for complete clearance. Many patients are quite prepared to tolerate minimal psoriasis such as that confined to knees and elbows. The inevitable tan which accompanies therapy is appreciated by all caucasians who regard it as a healthy sign. However, difficulties do arise when treating Indian and mongoloid races who do not wish to see their skin darken. Psoralens also sensitize the eyes to sunlight and as a precaution sunglasses must be worn for 8 hours after ingestion of psoralen and the patient advised to avoid sun exposure during this period.

Topical psoralen therapy has also been used in some centres with UVA but in our experience results have been poor and we have abandoned it.

Drug therapy

Etretinate

This drug (Tigason (Roche)) is one of a new family of retinoids which are derivatives of vitamin A and their use at present is solely confined to dermatology.

We have not found this drug of much benefit in the management of chronic plaque psoriasis but valuable in the management of acute pustular psoriasis (see below) and unstable plaque psoriasis with a tendency to pustulate. A maintenance dose of 0.25 mg/kg body weight is required.

Some centres use it prior to PUVA therapy and in a Finnish study prior administration of etretinate in a dose of 1.0 mg/kg significantly reduced subsequent PUVA dosage[15].

Other authorities however, disagree about this.

Side-effects include loss of hair in higher dose ranges and cracked lips. The drug is also teratogenic and female patients of child bearing age must take adequate contraceptive measures while on the drug and for a year afterwards.

Methotrexate

This is a very effective drug in controlling severe psoriasis. Unfortunately it has a serious side-effect of producing suppression of bone marrow and liver damage particularly in patients drinking alcohol. Patients therefore require careful monitoring.

In our practice most patients previously on methotrexate have been converted successfully to PUVA therapy. We now find it useful in short oral courses of 10 mg once weekly for 4–6 weeks in patients developing a relapse while receiving PUVA therapy.

Hydroxyurea

This is a useful drug and in a dose of 500 mg b.d. is a useful adjunct for in-patients not fully responding to other forms of therapy. It produces a dose-related rise in the mean corpuscular volume of RBCs which seems harmless but serves as an indicator that the patient is taking treatment.

We have not found it successful as a therapy on its own as it will not control severe psoriasis and is not necessary in cases responding to topical therapy except in the circumstances outlined above.

Pustular psoriasis

Localized form

Pustules appear on pre-existing plaques and in most cases this is due to previous treatment with tar or dithranol in a too high concentration. Therapy should be stopped and a bland application such as peanut ointment or zinc cream applied for a few days. If this fails then an all over application of a 1:4 dilution of betamethasone valerate (Betnovate RD (Glaxo)) for 2 days will usually remove the pustules and previous therapy can be re-instituted at half the original concentration.

Exanthematic form

This frequently follows streptococcal tonsillitis or upper respiratory tract infection. The patient is usually well and afebrile. Treatment with bland applications for a few days usually results in the pustules settling down to ordinary guttate psoriasis which can be treated as previously described.

Generalized pustular psoriasis (Von Zumbusch)

This can be a serious and life threatening disease and requires immediate in-patient admission and treatment.

Discrete areas of warm, painful erythema appear which may initially be mistaken for cellulitis. Multiple small, sterile pustules rapidly appear. Some coalesce to form lakes of sterile pus and pustules may sweep across the whole body in a series of waves. The patient is ill, usually febrile, and there is a leukocytosis and neutrophilia. Albumin seeps into the skin and the serum albumin and plasma volume may be drastically reduced. Hypocalcaemia and other electrolyte imbalance may be present.

Careful monitoring of renal function and electrolytes is essential.

The aetiology of the condition is unknown but it may follow cessation of corticosteroid therapy possibly for some other condition. It frequently arises *de novo*.

It is our practice to start these patients on a high dose of prednisolone of 80 mg/day for the average weight adult and to apply bland ointments to the skin. After 4 or 5 days the condition is usually vastly improved and PUVA therapy is introduced with UVA dosages beginning at half that recommended for plaque psoriasis and increments made at half the recommended rate also, on a twice weekly basis. Withdrawal of steroids is done gradually over a 3 week period by which time PUVA therapy will have taken effect. Fortunately the condition is rare and in the few cases we have treated we have given maintenance PUVA over 6 months reducing it to twice monthly treatments.

In one case where the condition recurred we used the same regimen and after PUVA gave a further 6 months therapy with etretinate 0.25 mg/kg. Long term maintenance therapy with PUVA or etretinate would seem at present to be the most suitable therapy for cases suffering frequent relapses. Methotrexate was also successful as maintenance therapy but has now largely been discarded because of side-effects as previously described.

Psoriasis of the nails

Treatment of this condition is unrewarding although some claim success with Dermojet infiltration of the skin overlying the nail base with triamcinolone.

CONCLUSION

It is salutary to reflect that the basic substances used in topical therapy of this condition have remained unaltered for over 50 years, and their mode of application and cosmetic acceptability have only recently been improved.

Little progress is likely to be made until basic research tells us more of the aetiology. The role of prostaglandins and the lipoxygenase enzyme pathway at present seem to be the most attractive lines of investigation but an open mind to all avenues is essential.

REFERENCES

1. Rea, J. N. (1976). Skin disease in Lambeth. *Br. J. Prevent. Soc. Med.*, **30**, 107–19
2. Cole, F. O. A. (1986). Personal communication
3. Marcusson, J., Moller, E. and Thyresson, N. (1976). Penetration of HLA-linked psoriasis predisposing gene(s). A family investigation. *Acta Dermato-Venereol.*, **56**, 453–5
4. Camp, R. D. R., Coutts, A. A., Greaves, M. W., Kay, A. B. and Walport, M. J. (1983). Responses of human skin to intradermal injection of leukotrienes C_4, D_4 and B_4. *Br. J. Pharmacol.*, **80**, 497–502
5. Allen, B. R. and Littlewood, S. M. (1983). The aetiology of psoriasis clues provided by benoxaprofen. *Br. J. Dermatol.*, **109**, Suppl. 25, 126
6. Seville, R. H. (1977). Psoriasis and stress. *Br. J. Dermatol.*, **97**, 297–302
7. Skoven, I. and Thormann, J. (1979). Lithium compound and treatment of psoriasis. *Arch. Dermatol.*, **115**, 1185–7
8. Ingram, J. T. (1953). The approach to psoriasis. *Br. Med. J.*, **2**, 591–6
9. Seville, R. H. (1975). Simplified dithranol treatment for psoriasis. *Br. J. Dermatol.*, **93**, 205–8
10. Runne, V. and Kunze, J. (1982). Short duration (minutes) therapy with dithranol for psoriasis. A new outpatient regimen. *Br. J. Dermatol.*, **106**, 135–9
11. Marsden, J. R., Coburn, P. R., Marks, J. and Shuster, S. (1983). Measurement of the response of psoriasis to short term application of anthralin. *Br. J. Dermatol.*, **109**, 209–18
12. Hindson, T. C., Diffey, B., Lawlor, F. and Downey, A. (1983). Dithranol-UV-A phototherapy (DUVA) for psoriasis: a treatment without dressings. *Br. J. Dermatol.*, **108**, 457–60
13. Armstrong, R. B., Leach, E. E., Fleiss, J. L. and Harber, L. C. (1984). Modified Goeckerman therapy for psoriasis. A two year follow-up of a combined hospital–ambulatory care program. *Arch. Dermatol.*, **120**, 3, 313–7
14. Wolff, K., Gschnait, F., Honigsmann, H., Konrad, K., Parrish, J. A. and Fitzpatrick, T. B. (1977). Phototesting and dosimetry for photochemotherapy. *Br. J. Dermatol.*, **96**, 1–12
15. Vaatainen, N., Hollmen, A. and Fraki, J. (1985). Trimethyl psoralen bath plus ultraviolet A combined with oral retinoid (etretinate) in the treatment of severe psoriasis. *J. Am. Acad. Dermatol.*, **12**, 52–7

INDEX

acne 1–25
  facial grades 4 (fig.)
  lesion formation 5
  psychological effects 2
  sunlight and 1
  treatment
    comedone removal 15
    cyst 19
    future 23–4
    immune complex reaction 15
    mild disease 15–16
    moderate disease 16–17
    non-responding patients 18–19
    oral: antibiotic 8–10, 16–17, 18, 20; dapsone 13; clofazimine 14; hormone 10–11, 17, 20; retinoids 11–13, 21–3
    scarring 19
    severe disease 16–18
    topical: antibiotic 6, 7–8; benzoyl peroxide 3–5, 7, 16; retinoic acid 6
acne keloid *see* folliculitis cheloidalis
acne necrotica 76
  miliaris 76
Actisorb 40
adrenaline 100, 101
Alphosyl-HC 130
Alprostadil 57
amitriptyline 100
Ancrod 57
angioedema 101–2
  hereditary 110–12
anti-androgen 7–8, 84
ascorbic acid 52
Aserbine 39
astemizole 99, 107

atherosclerosis 54
auto-haemotherapy 101
azelaic acid 7

bacitracin 69
bandage
  paste 47
  support 47–8, 50
benzoyl peroxide 5, 7, 40
benzyl-penicillin 77
Betadine 67, 88
betamethasone valerate (Betnovate RD) 133
Betnovate RD 133
brompheniramine maleate 99

calcium alginate (Sorbson, Kaltostat) 41
calcium gluconate 101
cephalexin 71, 77
cetrimide 39, 68
charcoal, activated (Actisorb) 40
chloramphenicol 6
chlorhexidine 66–7, 71, 91
chlorhexidine gluconate 39, 66–7
chlorhexidine–hydrocortisone–nystatin/(Nystaform-HC) 67
chlorhexidine–nystatin (Nystaform) 67
chlorocresol 39
cimetidine 100
cinnarizine 57
clindamycin 6, 81
clofazimine 60
cyclosporin-A 60
cyproheptadine 99, 107

danazol 112
Debrisan 40
dermabrasion 19
dermatitis artefacta, leg ulcers 36, 37 (fig.)
dermographism 101, 103–5, 107
dextranomer (Debrisan) 40
dithranol
   Ingram regime 127–8
   short contact 128
   +UVA (DUVA) 128–9
   staining prevention 129
dithranol–urea cream (Psoradrate) 130
doxantrazole 107
doxepin 100, 107

ecthyma 74, 75 (fig.)
eczema, bacterial infection of, 66, 88–91
Epoprostenol 57–8
erysipelas 77–9
erysipeloid 81–2
erythrasma 80, 81 (fig.)
erythromycin 6, 71, 77, 79–80, 82
ethanol
   with chlorhexidine 68
   with povidone–iodine 68
etretinate (Tigason) 131–2, 134
Eusol 39

fasciitis, necrotizing 80
Flamazine 68
flucloxacillin 71, 75, 89
folliculitis
   cheloidalis 76
   Gram-negative 18
   superficial 75–6
formalin, 1% aqueous 81
furunculosis 74–5
fusidic acid 68, 74, 80, 81

gangrene, postoperative bacterial 80
Geliperm 41–2
gentamicin 65, 68
Granuflex 41

H1 antagonists 94–5, 99–100, 101, 102–3
H2 antagonists 100, 103
heparin 101

hexachlorophane 68
Hibiscrub 67
Hibitane 66–7
Hioxyl 40
hives *see* urticaria
Hydroderm 69
hydrogen peroxide 40
hydroxyethylrutoside (Paroven) 52
hydroxyurea 132
hydroxyzine hydrochloride 99

imidazole 68, 80, 81
impetigo 72–4, 88
Inadine 88
indomethacin 103
infection, bacterial
   antibiotics
     contact allergy 65
     resistance 65
     steroid-antibiotic 66
     superinfection 65
     topical 68–70
   antiseptics 64, 66–7
inositol nicotinate 59
iodine granules (Iodosorb) 40, 88
Iodosorb 40, 88
isoniazid 85
isotretinoin 11–13, 17, 21–3, 84

Kaltostat 41
keratoderma blenorrhagicum 123
keratolysis, pitted 81, 82 (fig.)
ketotifen 100
Köbner phenomenon 117, 124
Köbner weals 109

lanolin 39
Lestreflex 47–8
Locoid 67

Malatex 39
medicament dermatitis 39
menaphthone 101
methotrexate 132
methyl testosterone 110
metronidazole 51–2
miconazole 68
Mupirocin 70
mycobacteria, atypical 86–7

INDEX

naftidrofuryl (Praxilene) 57
Naseptin 71
necrobiosis lipoidica 34, 59
neomycin 6, 69, 74
   contact sensitization 66
neomycin–bacitracin 74
neomycin–chlorhexidine (Naseptin) 71
nettle rash *see* urticaria
nicotinic acid 57
Nystaform 67
Nystaform-HC 67

oxatomide 100
oxypentifylline (Trental) 57

palmo-plantar pustulosis 123
parabens group, preservatives of 39
Paroven 52
penicillin 71, 79, 82
pit-viper venom (Ancrod) 57
polyacrylamide gel–agar hydrogel (Geliperm) 41–2
Polyfax 83
polymyxin B 69
polymyxin–bactracin (Polyfax) 83
Poroplast 47
post-phlebitic syndrome 45
povidone–iodine 39, 67, 71
   dressing (Inadine) 88
Praxilene 57
prednisolone 95, 110, 134
Prostacyclin (prostaglandin I_2) 57–8
prostaglandin 57–8
pseudofolliculitis 76
Pseudomonas aeruginosa infection 82–3
pseudomonic acid (Mupirocin) 70
Psoradrate 130
psoralen and UVA radiation (PUVA) 130–1, 134
psoriasis 115–35
   aetiology 116–17
   arthritis 115, 121–2, 124–5
   assessment 124–5
   erythrodermic 122–3
   guttate 122, 124, 129
   keratoderma blenorrhagicum 123
   nail
      hyperkeratosis 120
      onycholysis 121
      pitting 120
      treatment 134
   plaque 118–19, 125, 132
   pustular
      acute 132
      exanthematic 133
      generalized (von Zumbusch) 123, 133, 134
      localized 133
      palmo-plantar pustulosis 123
   treatment
      dithranol
         Ingram regime 127–8
         short contact 128; +UVA (DUVA) 128–9
      etretinate (Tigason) 131–2, 134
      hydroxyurea 132
      in-patient care 126
      methotrexate 132
      placebo role 26
      prednisolone 134
      psoralen and UVA radiation (PUVA) 130–1, 134
      rest 126
      scalp 130
      sedative 126
      steroids, topical 130
      tar and UVB radiation 129–30
PUVA therapy 130–1, 134
pyoderma gangrenosum 36

Quinocort 67
quinoline 67

ranitidine 100
Retin-A 15–16
retinoic acid 15–16
retinoid
   acne 11–12
   psoriasis 132
Roaccutane 7
rosaniline dye (Variclene) 40

scabies 103–4
Scherisorb 41
scratch trauma 103–4
Secure Forte 48
Sigvaris 50
silver 67–8
silver sulphadiazine 83

INDEX

sodium hypochlorite 39
Sorbsan 41
stanozolol (Stromba) 52–3, 112
staphylococcal scalded skin syndrome 74
Staphyloccous aureus
 carriage 70–1
 infection 71–2
steroid gel (Synalar Gel) 130
steroid–quinoline 89
steroid–tar cream (Alphosyl-HC) 130
stockings, elastic 50
Streptococcus pyogenes
 carriage 77
 infection 77
streptokinase–streptodornase (Varidase) 39
Stromba 52–3, 112
sulphadiazine (Flamazine) 68
sulphur 7
sulphur–salicyclic acid cream 80–1
suppurative hidradenitis 83–4
sycosis barbae 76
Synalar Gel 130
systemic lupus erythematosus 102–3

tar
 shampoo 130
 steroid–tar cream (Alphosyl HC) 130
 UVB radiation and 129–30
terbutaline 100
terfenadine 99–100, 107
tetracycline 6–7, 69–71, 74, 77, 82
Tigason 131–2
tranexamic acid 101, 110, 112
Trental 57
triamcinolone 134
trichomycosis axillaris 80–1
tricyclic anti-depressants 100
tuberculosis 85–6
Tubigrip 50

urticaria 93–114
 acute 93–5
  treatment 94–5
 angioedema associated 101
 aquagenic 107
 cholinergic 101, 104–5
  provocation test 105

 chronic 95–100
  differential diagnosis 95–6
  exacerbating factors 97
  hospital admission 99
  treatment 100–1
 cold 106–7
  desensitization 107
 physical
  cholinergic 101, 104–5, 107
  cold 106–7
  dermographism 107
  mixed patterns 107
 pressure 108–10
  Köbner weals 109
  mechanism 109
  treatment 110
 solar 107
 vasculitis and 102–3

ulcer, leg 29–61
 blood disorders 35
 cancer in 35
 debriding and cleansing 39–40
 dermatitis artefacta 36–7
 diabetic 33–4, 59
 diagnosis
  arterial (ischaemic) 33
  mixed 31
  venous 31–3
 dressing
  absorbent 40–2
  occlusive 42–3
 elderly 34
 infection
  cause 34–5
  complication 87–8
 ischaemic 53–8
  atherosclerosis 54
  investigations 55
  peripheral vascular disease 53–4
  treatment: amputation 55; analgesia 55; artery reconstruction 55; drugs 55, 56–7; hyperbaric oxygen 58; lumbar sympathectomy 55–6; wound cleansing 55
 medicament dermatitis 41
 necrobiosis lipoidica 34, 60
 pyoderma gangrenosum 36, 60
 tropical 34–5

INDEX

venous 43–53
  fibrin diffusion block therapy 44–5
  post-phlebitic syndrome 45
  treatment; compression 46–51; systemic drugs 51–3
  venous system 43–4

Variclene 40
Varidase 39
vasculitis, urticarial 102–3
Venosan 50

Viscopaste 47
von Zumbusch pustular psoriasis 123, 133, 134

Whitfield's ointment 80, 81

zinc
  leg ulcer 40, 52
  psoriasis 127
Zincaband 47
Zyderm 19